ENDORSEMENTS

"*Still Becoming* offers the freedom we've all been looking for. Steeped in scripture and wrapped in wisdom, each day's reading takes us one step closer to embracing a vital truth: our loving God created us to be healthy and whole. Prepare to breathe a deep sigh of relief, sisters. Hope is here!"

—Liz Curtis Higgs, best-selling author of *Bad Girls of the Bible*

"Are you tired of dieting? Gaining. Losing. Gaining. Losing. It can feel like a discouraging, demoralizing, and destructive collision course. Next comes guilt, followed by shame—and the cycle continues. In this honest, well-written, thirty-one-day devotional, Laura Acuña offers biblical, practical, and transformational help. This is the resource you've needed to begin embracing a grace-filled, joyful life."

—Carol Kent,
executive director of Speak Up Ministries; speaker;
author of *He Holds My Hand*

"When you read *Still Becoming*, you will meet a tender, faithful friend. That's who Laura Acuña is! In this wonderful devotional, she will give you the understanding of a trusted sojourner and the counsel of a very wise mentor! So read, enjoy, *become*, be blessed!!!"

—Jan Silvious, author of *Courage for the Unknown Season*

"Pause. Ponder. And gain PEACE as you process *Still Becoming: Hope, Help, and Healing for the Diet-Weary Soul*. Laura Acuña is a breath of fresh air and a voice of authenticity and wisdom."

—Pam Farrel,
author of 58 books including coauthor of the best-selling
Men Are Like Waffles, Women Are Like Spaghetti

"As a trained trauma counselor, I believe in this book. As someone who has struggled with disordered eating, I believe in this book. This devotional helps the reader interact not only with the truth of God's Word but also with the emotional struggles that underlie weight and body image. I would highly recommend this to my clients. Laura shares vulnerably from her own story and invites us to see God at work in our stories. Full of scripture and practical help, it is an incredible thirty-one-day healing journey that I want to invite everyone to join."

—Jennifer Hand,
author of *My Yes Is on the Table*; executive director of Coming Alive Ministries

"As an author, sitting for long periods of time has taken its toll on my weight and health. In *Still Becoming*, Laura Acuña shares her own story vulnerably, and her devotional makes you feel like you have the support and encouragement of a friend. What I love most about this book is the freedom it unlocks for the diet-weary soul. When you learn how to lose the guilt and shame, extra pounds seem to melt away with them!"

—**Anita Agers-Brooks**,
award-winning author of *Getting Through What You Can't Get Over*

"I am so excited for this book! Wow and wow! As a leader in the fashion industry, I see the damage women inflict on themselves by dieting and obsessing over the number on the scales. By giving up dieting for thirty-one days, a woman will now have a whole new outlook on her body because she will have done a deep dive into the *reasons* she continues on this roller coaster we call 'dieting.' This book is a must-read for most of the female population. I can't WAIT to give it to the women in my life."

—**Shari Braendel**,
founder of Style by Color and author of
Help Me Jesus, I Have Nothing to Wear!

"Have you struggled a lifetime with disordered eating and body issues? Do you ever just long to sit down with someone who understands all you have experienced, questioned, and fought to overcome? Oh, friend, let me graciously introduce you to author Laura Acuña and her newest book *Still Becoming*. Though I've read a fair amount of books on these subjects, I suspect I have never felt truly known and seen. Until now. Laura Acuña vulnerably shares her life with us, ultimately offering a better path to embracing the full and flourishing life God intended all along. And, it's not at the end of a diet. It's not a magic number on a scale. It is in true transformation from the inside out. Freedom. And that's why the butterfly on the cover is such a perfect visual for Laura's story. And perhaps yours and mine as well. Fill yourself with these thirty-one days of stories of inspiration and encouragement. And watch who you *become*."

—**Lucinda Secrest McDowell**,
award-winning author of *Soul Strong* and *Life-Giving Choices*

"I hardly have words for how much I love *Still Becoming*. Laura Acuña brings a breath of fresh hope for those who need to find peace with food and peace with themselves."

—**Vicki Heath**,
national director of First Place for Health

Laura Acuña

still
BECOMING

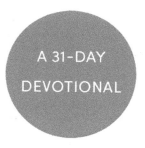

A 31-DAY
DEVOTIONAL

Hope, Help, and Healing
for the Diet-Weary Soul

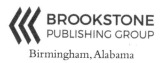

BROOKSTONE
PUBLISHING GROUP
Birmingham, Alabama

Still Becoming

Brookstone Publishing Group
An imprint of Iron Stream Media
100 Missionary Ridge
Birmingham, AL 35242
IronStreamMedia.com

Library of Congress Control Number: 2022911660

Cover design by Hannah Linder Designs

ISBN: 978-1-949856-79-8 (paperback)
ISBN: 978-1-949856-80-4 (e-book)

1 2 3 4 5—26 25 24 23 22

With love to my family: Pat, Patrick, Grant, Matthew, Angela, and Evelyn Grace. Thank you for cheering me on. Each one of you is a unique and precious treasure to me.

To Dr. Nicole K. Albertson, PsyD, and Amy Goldsmith, RDN, LDN: You taught me much of what I've shared in this book. Your expert guidance, patience, and grace helped set me free. Thank you for believing in me. I am eternally grateful.

And to all my Ezer-sisters with me in the struggle: Take heart. There is hope, help, and healing on the way. It is found only in the person of Jesus Christ.

WELCOME TO THE JOURNEY

I was tired. I was weary. *I was sick of it.*

I told God, "Lord, I would rather stay at the weight I am today than to keep losing and gaining it all back again."

I meant every word and syllable. It broke my heart to pray that prayer, but I was done.

I'd been dieting for almost five decades. For the life of me, I couldn't make my body cooperate with the scores and scores of diets I had attempted over all those long years.

It went like this: I lost the weight. I gained it back. Shame piled on. Lose. Gain. Shame. Repeat.

Sound familiar?

Because I have walked this journey, I know you are seeking answers too. Perhaps you have finally acknowledged the empty promises made by the dieting culture that have left you depleted and hopeless. You want to walk away from the burden of dieting but doing it would feel like giving up. Surrendering your dream to become healthy and whole seems *unbearable.*

I understand. I believed if I gave up dieting, it meant giving up my dream too. And I could not bear that, so I kept trying.

The good news is that, over time, God began challenging me to rethink my thinking about dieting, body image, and my unhealthy relationship with food.

What if I told you there's a better way?

When we're in the dieting mindset, we focus on untangling the way we eat, but we don't understand that what truly needs untangling is the way *we think.*

A few years ago, I mustered up the courage to give up dieting for good. I stepped off the crazy train—the one that continually promised me quick and permanent results but let me down every time. The one that played on my fears and counted on me gaining the weight back again so I could become *a lifetime member*. Can you relate?

After leaving dieting behind and learning to rethink my thinking, I surrendered my old way of looking at myself and the food issues that caused me so much pain. And, sweet friend, this is truly where the battle lies—in our mind and soul—*not on our plate*.

So, here's the truth. When I walked away from dieting, I gave up many things—but my dream wasn't one of them.

I've discovered that when we're free enough to treat our body and mind with care and respect, then *together* they will respond and heal.

And while I no longer suffer from disordered eating, I am still healing.

My thinking has been completely transformed, and my body is responding by becoming lighter, stronger, and healthier. I have come a long, long way on this journey, but I am *still becoming*.

I'm so grateful you have decided to bravely consider another way. What I am going to share with you over the next thirty-one days has completely changed my life. I believe with my whole heart it will change yours too.

I would like you to consider putting dieting on the back burner for our thirty-one days together. This is only a suggestion, but a dieting pause may help you focus on the daily content of this life-transforming message and put some of it into practice. Since we are in a grace-filled zone, you are completely free to choose what is best for you.

I am praying for redeemed, restored, and repaired hearts as we take the first brave steps toward thinking of our ourselves and our struggles in a brand-new way.

With so much love,

Laura

> *Be careful what you think,*
> *because your thoughts run your life.*
>
> Proverbs 4:23 NCV

HOW TO USE THIS BOOK

This devotional journal is a thirty-one-day journey through the lessons I've learned along the way. As we travel together, I will refer to any type of issues with food as *disordered eating*. This is a broad term that covers the variety of ways we may have an unhealthy relationship with food. We are not all the same, but we are in this *together*.

Still Becoming is divided into three sections: *My Story*, *Food for Thought*, and *Nourishment for Your Soul*.

Each day, I ask you to read the daily devotional and take part in a *Soul Fitness* exercise to strengthen your core. This is where our trust muscle is located. We're going to need to firm it up so we can stand strong and upright as we heal.

I've also included a daily prayer and space for you to journal your thoughts. I encourage you to go back every week or so to read what you have written previously and trace how you are growing day to day.

MY STORY

Most systems of weight loss fail because they don't live up to their promise: weight loss does not make people happy. Or peaceful. Or content. Being thin does not address the emptiness that has no shape or weight or name. Even a wildly successful diet is a colossal failure because inside the new body is the same sinking heart.

Geneen Roth

DAY 1

They dress the wound of my people
as though it were not serious.
"Peace, peace," they say,
when there is no peace.

Jeremiah 8:11

In Jeremiah's time, God's people believed false prophets and priests who promised peace, safety, and good things, but their trust was misplaced. Instead, the false prophets and priests made light of the people's brokenness and called them cured.

They declared peace, but there was no peace at all. In today's passage, Jeremiah is lamenting over God's people looking to false prophets instead of looking to the only One who can truly bring peace.

God's way meant repentance and turning toward His ways and His Word. Change was required. Instead, false teachers assured people that all would be fine. Of course, there was no true and lasting peace. Every single time God's people were caught up in putting their faith in anything other than God, chaos ruled.

I have done the same thing. I've placed my faith in the dieting industry with all its quackery. Instead of peace, I ended up in a cycle of debilitating defeat, and chaos ruled.

I misplaced my trust in programs and plans that made light of my real issues. Their interest lay in quick fixes they called victories, which consisted of *after pictures* that told nothing of what was really going on inside of a woman. These messages avoided the details involved in how she achieved her remarkable triumph. They didn't tell me how long she kept the weight off. Instead, they focused on success stories that once again simply promised me if I were skinny, I could feel free too.

It was in the fine print at the bottom of these so-called promises where they wrote a disclaimer, *results are not typical*, to cover themselves just in case the promise did not come true for me.

This billion-dollar industry, with my full permission, treated my wounds superficially and promised peace. But I found no such peace in what they delivered.

Even when I lost the weight—which I did many times—peace eluded me. I lived in terror I'd gain it back again. All my brokenness remained inside my body, regardless of its size.

My story is a long and winding tale, and friend, yours is too. It took a long time for me to understand I had placed my trust in all the wrong places.

Thankfully, God is so incredibly patient, as He kindly waits for us to turn back to Him. He knows how we are. We chase after quick fixes and immediate results. Yet, He offers so much more through Jesus Christ, our Savior.

When Jesus healed people, He healed them of their infirmities, both body and spirit, but He also restored a sense of belonging and took away their shame. He does the same for us, I know this from experience.

I gave up dieting and embraced healing. Will you join me on the journey?

SOUL FITNESS: Strengthening Your Core

When you consider giving up dieting for thirty-one days, does it feel scary? Journal your thoughts as we begin our journey together. Write down your apprehension, excitement, anxiousness—whatever emotions you are feeling. Remember, you are still becoming.

PRAYER

Lord, I am feeling a variety of emotions as I begin this thirty-one-day devotional. I am afraid to hope there might be a way to walk away from the dieting mindset without giving up my healthy body dream. Please light my path. Please encourage me along the way. Please give me courage to see this through. Amen.

7/29/2023

Food, weight body image &
self worth have always
been an issue for me.
To lay that all down
and just be "loving kind
and gentle with myself ♡
"Amazing". ♡

DAY 2

As Scripture says, "Anyone who believes in
him will never be put to shame."

Romans 10:11

My shame story began when I was eleven. I entered seventh grade at five feet tall and weighed one hundred pounds, but by the time I left junior high, my weight doubled. Yes, you read that correctly. In the brief span of only a few years, I gained over one hundred pounds.

As a woman, I know you do not need me to detail how traumatic this was for me. Gaining so much weight in such a short amount of time was like a bomb going off in my eleven-year-old life. *Everything changed.*

I have a vivid memory from when I was twelve. Believing I was out of earshot, a well-meaning relative fretted to my mother, "Oh, what a shame. Laura Anne was such a pretty girl. What a terrible shame."

Honestly, my relative was telling the truth for the most part and she never meant to hurt me. The experience of gaining so much weight was truly a terrible shame. Even so, my young ears didn't hear "*it* is a shame." Instead, I interpreted her comments as "*she* is a shame" and I believed it.

In 1970, no one knew what to do with a little girl who gained one hundred pounds in the seventh grade. Little was known about disordered eating in those days. In sincerely trying to help me, my mother took me to a local weight loss program. From that day on, I lived in a love/hate relationship with all things concerning dieting. I began forcing my body to do something it wasn't created to do.

My body went from being the fun part of me that ran, skipped, danced, twirled, and played, to becoming my sworn enemy. I began to disconnect from and loathe the physical part of me.

We often believe the words *guilt* and *shame* have the same meaning, but that's not true. Guilt says, "You've *made* a mistake." Shame says, "You *are* a mistake."

Do you hear the difference? Healthy guilt, prompted by the Holy Spirit, pushes you toward repentance and restoration. Shame pushes you toward despair and self-condemnation. It is not from your God.

My internal dialogue was filled with harsh words toward myself, and if that wasn't tragic enough, the dieting culture gave me even more ammo.

Maybe you'll recognize some of these shame statements:

- I am being bad.
- I am cheating.
- I need to starve myself all week because I ate too much.
- I can't have what everyone else is having because I'm fat.
- I must hide parts of my body because they are ugly.

Do you hear the harshness in these condemning thoughts?

The voice of shame, originating from Satan, whom I call *The Shamer*, tells you you're defective. He started telling me that lie when I was just eleven years old. He convinces you that your only hope of restoration is to weigh a certain number and look a certain way.

Shame is expensive—it cost me so much. But I think what really impacted me most was my completely unbiblical belief about God and His intentions toward me. And the most heartbreaking belief of all? For far too long, I thought the voice of The Shamer *belonged to my heavenly Father.*

Thankfully, as my faith grew, and I learned to line my thinking up with God's Word, I eventually recognized the sweet voice of my Savior. The way He spoke to me was in stark contrast to the condemning voice I had been listening to for so long. Jesus's voice was full of grace, kindness, and love. The more I recognized God and paid attention to what He said about me, the more the voice of The Shamer steadily became silent.

Just as the voice of my Savior is in stark contrast to the voice of The Shamer, so are His ways. The Shamer brings severe restrictions and legalism regarding food and how we relate to our bodies.

But listen to Jesus's way . . .

Are you tired? Worn out? Burned out on religion? Come to me. Get away with me and you'll recover your life. I'll show you how to take a real rest. Walk with me and work with me—watch how I do it. Learn the unforced rhythms of grace. I won't lay anything heavy or ill-fitting on you. Keep company with me and you'll learn to live freely and lightly. (Matthew 11:28–30 MSG)

Anyone ready to learn the *unforced rhythms of grace*? Let's go!

SOUL FITNESS: Strengthening Your Core

Have you mistaken the voice of The Shamer for the voice of God? Journal all the areas in your life where shame has seeped in. Now contrast your shame experiences against the life-giving words of Matthew 11:28–30. What are the differences?

PRAYER

Heavenly Father, I've been listening to The Shamer for too long. Please help me line up my thoughts with your Word. I want to readily recognize your voice when you speak to me. Thank you for offering me truth and grace. Amen.

"Accident" "She's not pretty"
Outta the house, hurt & pain,
choosing others, Hate and
anger, you're a mistake, never
enough ;:(: you should be
in church

DAY 3

The accumulated sorrows of your exile
will dissipate.
I, your God, will get rid of them for you.
You've carried those burdens long enough.

Zephaniah 3:18 MSG

I've done a little research on the typical woman who suffers from disordered eating. We are all different with vastly unique experiences—but, as disordered eating is studied, a common personality emerges. I'm paraphrasing the work of Dr. Anita Johnston, who is a recognized expert on disordered eating in women.

The typical woman who suffers from disordered eating picked up early in life that her emotions needed to be tamped down, hidden away and silenced. She often felt she was too much and not enough all at the same time. Many report they had a pervasive sense of not fitting in, of not seeing things the way others did, and of being a misfit.

As she is naturally intuitive and sensitive, this posed a problem for her. Her family, for one reason or another, did not appreciate her sensitivity, perspective, and honesty. She often received the message—sometimes nonverbal—that her outspoken, questioning behavior was not acceptable.

Keeping the peace was the priority. There was to be no rocking the family boat. So, she did what anyone with limited choices would do—she complied, silenced herself, denied her intuition, and voluntarily dimmed her light. She did it by turning to food for comfort and dieting for some measure of control.

The adolescent experience described in Dr. Johnston's words above is part of my long and winding story. Tears flowed when I discovered the truth regarding the typical woman with disordered eating. Until I learned differently, I thought I was the only one.

I long believed the attributes God designed into me—my thin skin, curiosity, intuition, and ability to read between the lines—were flaws instead of gifts. Oh, how The Shamer distorts what is good!

Friend, my deepest hope, now that we are on the third day of our time together, is that you, too, understand you are not alone. As children, we had little in the way of choices. It was reasonable for us to adapt to the expectations demanded of us. *But we aren't children anymore.* Our childhood coping mechanisms are obsolete.

Instead of helping us to survive, these coping mechanisms now threaten to keep us from becoming our true selves—the women God created us to be.

For most of my life I have been a world-class stuffer. I didn't feel safe expressing my genuine emotions. If I were angry or sad, I slapped a big smile over my hurting heart and denied what was going on under the surface. *I am just fine*, became my masked persona.

As an Olympic-level people pleaser, I couldn't stand the thought of anyone being upset with me. So, I often played along and pacified the person who was angry. I don't recommend this way of relating to others. It's not honest, even when presented with a smile.

Some of us turn to food when negative emotions rise, and we are uncomfortable. Instead, when emotions flood in, can we practice a pause and turn to Jesus?

I know that sounds like the proverbial Sunday school answer, but it's more than that. Consider the deeper meaning behind the following Scripture: "Trust in him at all times, O people; pour out your heart before him; God is a refuge for us. Selah" (Psalm 62:8 ESV). The Hebrew word *Selah* occurs between verses or paragraphs in parts of the Old Testament, often in the Psalms, indicating a pause for contemplation. It means "to stop and listen—to pause and praise."

When we learn to pour our hearts out to God first, instead of stuffing our emotions, childhood coping mechanisms aren't needed anymore. Let this soak in. You've carried this burden long enough. Let the Lord get rid of your childhood behaviors once and for good. Praise His name.

SOUL FITNESS: Strengthening Your Core

Today, when you feel negative emotions arise, consciously decide to turn to God first, before stuffing them or turning to the fridge. Build a repertoire of ways you can soothe yourself when you are feeling upset. Take a walk. Go for a drive. But whatever action you take, experience your true feelings. Stop and listen. Pause and praise. You will feel so much better than if you stuffed it all. You can be honest and real before God.

PRAYER

Father, thank you for being a refuge for me in times of trouble. I want to learn to trust that my feelings will not take me out, but stuffing them will. Help me find more ways to soothe myself than with food. Remind me that I have a variety of healthier choices when negative emotions arise. I'm ready for this burden to be lifted. Amen.

DAY 4

God, pick up the pieces.
Put me back together again.
You are my praise!

Jeremiah 17:14 MSG

As we allow ourselves to feel the emotions we have avoided for so long, stories will emerge from our past that can advise us on our *why*. Why are my feelings ramped up? Why do I turn to food for comfort and calm? Why did this happen in the first place?

Our stories are important to remember and process so we can find pieces to the puzzles of our lives. We need to make sense of why we futilely chose food to fix all our broken places and hide part, or even all, of ourselves away.

When recollections pop up, it's important to pause and ask God what we need to glean from our past experiences. All along the way, He is intimately involved in our healing. He sits with us in both our joyful and heartbreaking stories.

We can trust Him to be with us as we examine the truth of our story and can also trust He will help us understand how our past impacts us today.

I've heard the Lord referred to as a *Divine Archaeologist*. What a perfect name for our Healer. Archaeologists are sent to ruins of past civilizations to dig into the sites and discover important stories of what happened there. They use tiny brushes and picks as they carefully search for artifacts buried under the ground. I am amazed at their patience, just as I'm in awe of God's endurance and gentleness with us.

If we allow Him, the Divine Archaeologist will gently and tenderly excavate the layers of our pasts. He will do it slowly and sweetly, taking great care not to injure. It takes a while, but the treasures He unearths in us are worth the wait.

Finally, underneath all the dust, dirt, and grime of our lives, after gently scraping and digging, God brings the broken parts of our story out into the light and washes them clean. What was found may be broken—but He redeems, restores, and repairs. And unlike a human archaeologist, *He has all the pieces.* He can put us completely back together again. Our own uncovered story helps us understand how the past influenced our present.

Friend, for a long time now, I have invited God to excavate the layers of my life. Unburying the past has proven a crucial part of my recovery. And since I am *still becoming*, the excavating will continue, probably until He calls me home. I'm okay with that. The more He and I dig together, the more I learn about myself. But more importantly, *the more I learn about Him.*

I can tell you with certainty that without going back, you cannot move forward. If we hide from the truth of our lives—if we bury and stuff the past—we will never be healthy and whole.

In order to heal, you must ask God to help you to find and understand the missing pieces of your story. And when you do, make sure you look back on your experiences with self-compassion and curiosity. As you gain clarity and understanding, the journey toward healing moves forward.

SOUL FITNESS: Strengthening Your Core

Today, ask God to excavate the layers of your past. Ask Him to clarify questions when memories pop up. Sit in stillness and listen. You may need to process revelations with a trusted friend or a counselor. Openness is such a brave step on the healing path.

PRAYER

God, I am ready to look back so I can move forward. I know some of the memories will be painful. Thank you for promising to stay close to me when I am hurting. I want to be healthy and whole. I am committing to do what it takes to become free. Amen.

DAY 5

Therefore do not worry or be anxious
(perpetually uneasy, distracted), saying,
"What are we going to eat?" or
"What are we going to drink?" or
"What are we going to wear?"

Matthew 6:31 AMP

I honestly believe there are no bad foods. Yes, some foods we need to limit, or eat wisely, but they aren't bad—unless we're talking about deep-fried cheesecake. That is *definitely bad*, though I imagine it tastes oh so good. LOL

In the past, my disordered brain stayed on alert, policing what I put in my mouth. The scrutinizing began anytime I opened the fridge, packed my lunch, planned family meals, or opened a menu. I felt terrorized and exhausted.

I evaluated everything I ate. *Am I being good? Am I being bad?*

On top of that, *friends of the food police* kept changing the rules, which only added to the craziness. One diet plan told me fruit was *free* and I could eat as much as I wanted. Another proclaimed fruit was *bad* and to be eaten sparingly.

Various low-carb diets encouraged me to eat butter, bacon, and mayonnaise—others only allowed a teaspoon of olive oil a day. Some plans required strict compliance, meaning one slip ruined everything. If I ate something not on the program—like an evil carb—it was back to the beginning. And then there were the diets that offered *cheat days*, which are among the most counterproductive ways to develop a healthy relationship with food. *My goodness.* No wonder I felt confused.

When I was in my early twenties, I signed up for a dieting center program. I paid a lot of money for them to tell me I could eat only six hundred and fifty calories a day.

Every day, I was allowed one apple, a few hard-boiled eggs, a half cup of vegetables and their special supplements. That was it. Anything that didn't make the list was bad. Skinny was the goal. I could get healthy later. I lost a lot of weight on this program, but I was starving and miserable.

Eventually, my body had enough of the way I treated it and stopped losing weight—even when I ate so little food. At my weekly weigh-in, the woman who ran the center evaluated my food diary and concluded that I had been bad. Of course, she did. The diet worked. I didn't.

After careful scrutiny, she determined my weight loss plateau was coming from the pink sugar substitute I put in my black coffee. She warned me, "This has a *trace of sugar*, so it must be the tiny culprit." In an act of super food-policing, she took my fake sugar away. How heartless!

Of course, my weight boomeranged back. My body tried to save me from myself by lowering my metabolism.

You see, God created our physical selves to protect us, even when we abuse them. Had I stayed on that tortuous diet, I would have lost more weight after beating my body into submission—but at what cost? How might my physical health have suffered while I tried to appease the food police? How much unnecessary anxiety might my mind have endured? At that time, freedom felt so elusive to me. I had been living under the weight of food obsessions since I was eleven years old.

The only thing I knew was to keep hunting for the perfect diet for me. I didn't understand I had an emotional and spiritual problem that needed an emotional and spiritual answer. It took time, but finally and with mustard seed faith at first (Matthew 17:20), I turned away from the world's diet mantras and moved toward healing for my mind and soul.

Little by little, and with help from my beloved therapist, Nicole, and brilliant dietician, Amy, I fired the food police and all their friends. It was scary, but when I took the first step, I found firm ground beneath my feet. I sought skilled and gentle helpers to guide me—there's no shame in that. The professionals I worked with infused the entire experience with much, much needed grace.

Girls, we honor our bodies by eating whole, nutritious food *most of the time*. Do you hear the absence of legalism in that statement? When we rightly view food as *just food*, understanding God provides it to fuel the bodies He designed, we learn to make choices that are best for us. This includes how much and what food *we choose* to eat.

Also remember, God gave us food for pleasure too—and treating ourselves occasionally is *normal*. We shouldn't go into a tailspin and starve ourselves the next day when we've enjoyed a treat. Accept your normalcy and move on.

I've discovered if I eat three healthy meals a day and snacks if needed, I am satiated. I am calm. And when I'm calm, I no longer obsess about food.

When we connect to our bodies and emotions, then listen to them both, food falls into its rightful place in our lives. The emotional charge disappears.

Listen, it doesn't matter what the food police tells you. Freedom, my sisters, is not a number on the scale.

I fired the food police and God brought peace and health to my body, mind, and spirit. Isn't it time for you to take that healthier step for yourself?

SOUL FITNESS: Strengthening Your Core

Are you ready to fire the food police? Make a list of all their offenses and commit to letting them go.

PRAYER

Lord, your Word tells me you are not a God of disorder but of peace (1 Corinthians 14:33). Bring order to my disorder. Bring peace to my chaos. Bring freedom to my body and soul. Amen.

DAY 6

Do you not know that your bodies are temples of the
Holy Spirit, who is in you, whom you have received from
God? You are not your own; you were bought at a price.
Therefore honor God with your bodies.

1 Corinthians 6:19–20

I hated my body. The hatred hinged on two deeply held and rigid beliefs. They were both so hard to give up. One, I've already confessed. I viewed my body as a sworn enemy. Two, I also believed if I accepted my body, I'd have to accept being overweight for the rest of my life.

Translated: If I love my body, I am admitting defeat.

Again, it all comes down to how we think. My tangled thoughts of dieting and body image were my security blanket. I believed if I even entertained liking my body, I would give up my dream.

But, as I began my journey, I found my long-held beliefs were an obstacle to my progress. My false perceptions were in the way. It wasn't easy—but they had to go.

For me to be free from disordered eating, I had to work *with* my body—not *against* it. I had to learn how to trust what it told me. We can't hate our body into being healthy. We will not respect something we loathe, and we can't love what we don't trust.

After decades of disconnection and disdain, trust seemed impossible, and love unthinkable. But nothing is impossible with God.

Over time, I learned to love and trust my body. This may sound unbelievable, but it's true.

It was surprising to discover I could love my body and yet not feel satisfied with where I was in that moment. I learned to say to myself, *I am healing. I am still becoming. There is grace.*

I can cultivate a healthy relationship with the body I have today and not wait for the thinner one I will have tomorrow. For me, the secret to loving and trusting my body is to treat it well and watch how it responds. At the beginning, I had much to learn and so much to let go of, but the fruit of this work has been remarkable.

According to a recent study by the National Institutes of Health, 91 percent of women report they are unhappy with their bodies. We know this reflects our culture and the toxic messages we have received over a lifetime.

This is not the message of Scripture, though. In Psalm 139 we are told that we are fearfully and wonderfully made. In 1 Corinthians 6:19, Paul makes a dramatic claim. He says our bodies are temples of the Holy Spirit. I have often felt convicted by this verse, and for good reason.

Repentance is required when we've abused our bodies. There is no healing without owning our sin.

When we view today's verse through the lens of grace, can we also hear it saying to us that this body we are walking around in is *where the Holy Spirit dwells*? It is the house of our eternal soul. But do we understand this? *Really?*

If so, can we agree that God wouldn't house His Spirit or our souls in a dysfunctional, loathsome dwelling? And how should we respond to the counter-culture message God's Word sends us?

Sister, there will be no lasting peace without learning to love and trust the bodies God gave you and me.

SOUL FITNESS: Strengthening Your Core

Journal prompt: Dear Body, you are worth loving because . . .

List all the ways your body is worth loving. Start with ten things your body helps you do.

PRAYER

Dear Jesus, thank you for creating my miraculous body. Help me to reconnect with my physical self and treat it with honor and respect. It's hard to imagine loving something I've been at war with for so long, but I'm ready to try. Amen.

DAY 7

*Make allowance for each other's faults, and forgive anyone
who offends you. Remember, the Lord forgave you,
so you must forgive others.*

Colossians 3:13 NLT

There is no healing without forgiveness. Our outdated coping mechanisms are a response to painful and unmanageable parts of our stories.
Once we come to terms with this fact, we'll have some releasing to do. It's
hard to lay down the unhealthy ways we cope, without clearing away the
rubble of unforgiveness.

Intentionally or not, boyfriends, parents, friends, and spouses might
have said and done hurtful things to us. Both deliberate and accidental
wounds cut deep, and emotional memories can live on for a lifetime.

The problem is, if we stay stuck in unforgiveness, we remain victim-
ized by the one who hurt us. We can't move forward. If we're going to
find victory over the hurts that drove us to use food as an escape, we must
resolve the past.

You've likely heard this familiar statement: *Unforgiveness is like drink-
ing poison yourself and waiting for the other person to die.* This description
creatively explains how an unwillingness to release emotional baggage
is toxic to our own souls. The Shamer likes to tell us we are justified

in withholding forgiveness—after all, the perpetrator hurt us. But if we entertain his deception, Satan has us right where he wants us. His plan is to convince us that God didn't actually say we must forgive *everyone*. If we buy into The Shamer's lies, he wins.

I know forgiveness may seem daunting, if your hurts are deep and soul wounding—especially when abuse is involved. If this is part of your story, I am so sorry. I hope you know our grace-filled and patient Father understands forgiveness will be a long-term process for some of us. And He sees you and loves you, no matter how long it takes.

We can confidently trust God with our shattered hearts. He is true to His character and will never ask us to do anything He will not give us the power to see us through.

As you begin the hard work of healing, remember there are many misconceptions about what it means to extend forgiveness to another. Here are important truths to understand:

- *We are not letting the other person off the hook.* Forgiveness begins with righteous anger and acknowledges the offense was wrong and hurtful. Releasing unforgiveness lets us off the hook. We become free.

- *We do not need the person's involvement or cooperation to forgive them.* The object of our forgiveness does not need a voice in the conversation between us and God. This protects our tender hearts and means that even if the person is deceased, forgiveness can still happen.

- *Forgiveness does not mean reconciliation.* Restoring a relationship is a separate discussion and decision between God and you.

- *We will never forget.* When we forgive, we don't experience holy amnesia where the memory goes away. Only God forgives and forgets. When we release unforgiveness, we also give up the right for revenge and refuse to let old hurts control us any longer.

Forgiveness frees us emotionally so we can risk trusting again. We need to forgive out of obedience and trust in our loving Father, who knows what is best for His children. When we do, we discover the relief and inner peace that never lasted with food.

But there is one more reason forgiveness is important. Every human being has a desperate need for forgiveness and grace; after all, no one is perfect or mistake-free. So, how on earth can we withhold from others what we so deeply desire for ourselves when we mess up—understanding, mercy, compassion, patience, and grace?

When you forgive, you will be surprised to find the gift isn't for the offender, but for you. And if you are like me, you will also discover that after deciding to release your anger, food's hold on you isn't nearly as strong.

SOUL FITNESS: Strengthening Your Core

Sweet friend, are you harboring unforgiveness? Carve out some time to chat with God today, using the prayer below. Give yourself the gift of relief and peace.

PRAYER

Heavenly Father, today I come before you to ask, "Search me, God, and know my heart; test me and know my anxious thoughts. See if there is any offensive way in me, and lead me in the way everlasting" (Psalm 139:23–24). I am ready to do the hard work of forgiving. Thank you for your patience and compassion with me. Amen.

DAY 8

Do not be conformed to this world, but be transformed
by the renewal of your mind.

Romans 12:2 ESV

Before stepping onto the healing path of becoming free, I pictured myself as a young girl living inside of a dark cocoon. While it felt familiar and safe, as time went on, I experienced a nagging sense that it was time to break out of what kept me bound. But I didn't know how.

Satan, God's number one enemy and ours, wants us to believe we belong inside a cocoon. He wants us to think we deserve darkness. But those are more of his lies. We were made to live out in the light, where Jesus is.

Romans 12:2 tells us we are transformed when we renew our minds. The Greek translation of the word *transformed* is *metamorfoo*, which means "to be changed into something completely new. Permanently changed."

Metamorfoo describes the process by which what is happening on the *inside*, becomes evident on the *outside*. This is where our English word *metamorphosis* originated.

The Greek translation of the word *renew* means "to make new" or "moving from one stage into a more developed one. Continual renewal—a renewing process."

Romans 12:2 perfectly describes how God works to mature and heal us when we are ready to get well. We undergo a continual process of renewal, moving from one stage to a more developed one, when we align our actions with His will. What is happening on the inside of us is eventually revealed on the outside, visible to others.

Once transformed, we become a new creation—permanently changed. The dieting culture makes a similar promise. There's only one difference: they can't deliver.

When we think of metamorphosis, we often envision a butterfly. And when we think of a butterfly, we imagine a cocoon. But do we give much thought to exactly what goes on inside?

Inside the cocoon where no one else can see, this creature is becoming her true, mature self—exactly what her Creator designed her to be. She will not end up being just a better version of a caterpillar. She will become an entirely new creation.

At first, the changes aren't clear to the outside world. Only the caterpillar and her Creator know what is going on as she transforms. But once the metamorphosis is complete, the butterfly breaks free and flies.

Friend, our God is willing to do the same for us. He can change us from the inside out. We must invite Him into the process and exercise patience while He spends the time necessary to transform us into the free and beautiful being He desires. And we must understand that this work is invisible on the outside—at first, even to us.

When you make the decision to rely on God regarding your food choices and body image, your transformation will only be visible between you and your Creator. Only the two of you will see the changes taking place. That's okay.

I've learned there is a time when it's safe and necessary to exist inside the cocoon, but we are not meant to stay there. The cocoon is a place of growth and change—not a place to hide and lay dormant. The only way out is *transformation*.

There is one more thing I want to share with you about transformation. Contrary to popular dieting beliefs, you can be transformed and set free in your mind and spirit while your body is still healing. In other words, you can experience freedom before you *ever lose a pound*. For some of us, this is how it works. Ponder this idea and we'll discuss it more tomorrow.

SOUL FITNESS: Strengthening Your Core

Consider how God may be healing you on the inside even before you or others see evidence of it on the outside. Journal anything you notice about your thinking or how things may be changing. Celebrate each time you notice something new.

PRAYER

God, I want to become something completely new—permanently changed. Help me avoid conforming to the patterns of my culture, but instead teach me to conform to your Word. As I take my first steps on the healing path, show me how my thinking can transform. Thank you, Father. Amen.

DAY 9

So we're not giving up. How could we! Even though on the outside
it often looks like things are falling apart on us, on the inside,
where God is making new life, not a day goes
by without his unfolding grace.

2 Corinthians 4:16–18 MSG

What you weigh has nothing to do with how free you are. I know, I know. Our whole lives, we've been led to believe a free woman is a skinny one, but that's just another lie.

If you think about it, you likely know women who are at their ideal weight—whatever that is—but are still consumed with thoughts of food and body image. They may not have an ounce of fat on them, but they are in bondage.

My entire life I believed freedom meant skinny. I don't know why I held onto that fable. From my own experience, I knew that every time I reached my goal weight, anxiety and obsession haunted me. I just wore smaller clothes while I worried.

A few years ago, I was invited to attend a weekend retreat for women who suffer with food and body image strongholds. I'd never taken part in anything like this event. It was the first time I realized my issues were not only emotional and physical, but spiritual. From the moment I arrived, the Lord began dealing with my wrong thinking regarding food and freedom.

The women who attended came in all shapes, ages, backgrounds, and sizes. It felt glorious gathering with others who struggled like I did.

When I took my seat at the first session of the retreat, I sat near a woman who by our culture's standards had quite a bit of weight to lose. I immediately started judging her. My heart felt empathy, but I judged all the same.

Based on what she looked like, I determined she had just started her healing journey and had a long, long way to go until she found freedom. From my perspective, this meant when she reached her ideal weight. I concluded she struggled with the worst possible bondage, until I met her and heard her story.

I soon realized God was dealing with my wrong thinking and was about to transform my broken mind. I was becoming. So was my new friend.

I found out this sister had been on the healing journey for a long time. She no longer used food to soothe her hurting heart. Many pounds had already melted away, making her lighter, stronger, and healthier. Though her body still needed further healing, I began to understand that *she was free. I was not.*

This revelation blew me away. I felt truly humbled and repentant for my judgmental thoughts. Understanding this eye-opening truth about deliverance served me well on my own healing journey.

Freedom lies in our mind and spirit. It is a work of God and has nothing to do with food or weight. Our weight will fluctuate—our freedom will not.

I realized this truth in my own life when the quarantine for COVID-19 began. I compared it to being confined in my home during a blizzard.

During a big snowstorm I followed my instincts and stocked up on all my favorite comfort foods. I spent my days making rich stews and pot roasts, cookies, and other special treats. It was over the top, trust me.

But, in the early days of the quarantine, I came to the stunning realization that even though we were confined and anxious about the virus, I no longer turned to food to cope. I made trips to the grocery store for our staple items—not my favorite goodies. It never even crossed my mind to buy my comfort foods. At long last, turning to healthier ways of dealing with stress and heartache came naturally.

I've learned that disordered thinking leads to disordered eating, and when the first part is transformed, the rest follows. We aren't giving up our dream to live lighter, stronger, and healthier, but the truth is, we can be free before we ever lose a pound.

SOUL FITNESS: Strengthening Your Core

Spend some time pondering today's devotion. Do you agree that freedom from disordered eating and negative body image has nothing to do with what you weigh? Why or why not?

PRAYER

Lord, I want to be free. I acknowledge it's sometimes easier to just keep living the way I am instead of dealing with how I ended up in bondage. Please give me the courage to stay the course and to trust you with my brokenness. Please help me remember the goal is healing—not a number on the scale. Amen.

FOOD FOR THOUGHT

You will never cease to be the most amazed person at what God has done for you on the inside.

Oswald Chambers

DAY 10

*Finally, brothers and sisters, whatever is true, whatever is noble, what-
ever is right, whatever is pure, whatever is lovely, whatever
is admirable—if anything is excellent or praiseworthy—think about
such things. Whatever you have learned or received
or heard from me, or seen in me—put it into practice.
And the God of peace will be with you.*

Philippians 4:8–9

How much time do you spend thinking about food? What about your body? Other people's perceptions of what you eat and how you look? These and other questions are important for us to consider if we want to become who we are meant to be.

- Do you ruminate over what you ate yesterday and what you will not eat today?
- Do you spend too much time picking out what you will wear each day and how you will look?
- Are you fixated on a certain number on the scale?
- Do you go to bed at night and wake up in the morning thinking about food, your body, and what others think of you?

It's exhausting just writing this down, and I've only provided a partial list. Yet, this was me and my thoughts.

Can you imagine clearing your brain of these concerns? Try to picture yourself with enough mental space to think about the things that God wants to do in and through your life.

Women on the dieting roller coaster spend an inordinate amount of precious time thinking about food and body image. Obsessive and recurring thoughts become so normal we don't even realize what we are telling ourselves. And of course, shame's tentacles worm their way in and create quite another distraction.

The problem is, when we ruminate and worry over our body and food obsessions, there's little space left over to pursue the things of God. In Philippians 4:8–9, Paul tells us the beneficial things God wants our minds to dwell on. These praiseworthy thoughts, when put into practice, will bring us God's peace.

You will be surprised to find that when you reconnect with your body, honor what it is telling you, and respond to what it needs, your thinking will be transformed. As you move from restriction to nourishment, move your body for improved mental and physical health, trust your hunger cues to tell you when to eat and when to stop, your brain will calm down. You will experience peace. It will not happen overnight, but it will happen.

Not too long ago, the concept of freeing up brain space felt foreign to me. I couldn't imagine how I might discover freedom from the mental tyranny I had lived under since I was a little girl. This was one reason I sought healing. Anxiety, worry, and obsession exhausted me.

As God began healing me, I noticed I went days without obsessing over my body and food. Honestly, it was shocking. As my mind settled down, I found I had more bandwidth to think creatively and peacefully. As my mind freed, so did my life. I took more risks, stepped way out of my shame-filled comfort zone, and left the tyranny of fear behind.

A food-and-body-image obsessed brain will keep you from the things God has called you to do and from becoming who He has created you to be. Take the risk. With each step on the healing path and as more truth is revealed to you, freedom will come. You will be more present with your family and friends and more able to serve God and care for others. The toxic thinking that has terrorized you for so long will become history.

When you clear your brain space from obsessing over a number on the scale and all that comes with it, you will have more space for J.O.Y. Jesus. Others. You.

SOUL FITNESS: Strengthening Your Core

What would it look like if you experienced a day where you no longer filled your brain space with thoughts of food, your body, and all that comes along with them? How would you feel?

PRAYER

Father, my mind is filled with thoughts that keep me from living the life you planned for me. I know I am in bondage to thoughts about my body: how it looks, what I feed it, and what it weighs. I am exhausted and depleted, but your Word tells me that if I think on the things You want to fill my mind with, I will have peace. Help me put this into practice. Help me learn to think in a new way—one that aligns with the plan and purpose you have for my life—one that helps me become as you desire. Amen.

DAY 11

Then we will no longer be immature like children. We won't be tossed and blown about by every wind of new teaching. We will not be influenced when people try to trick us with lies so clever they sound like the truth.

Ephesians 4:14 NLT

Nearly twenty years ago I attended a Women of Faith conference in Washington D.C. One of the speakers was Jan Silvious who shared a message based on her book *Big Girls Don't Whine*. The title captured me, and her wise words opened my eyes to something I had never considered. I remember sitting there taking in her teaching, feeling as if I were the only one in the arena.

Jan challenged us to grow up and become *Big Girls*—mature women in Christ. With her typical grace and humor, Jan described the disadvantages of remaining a little girl into our adulthood. It was then I realized I still possessed many little girl behaviors, long past the age when they were appropriate. Looking back, I'm sure everyone in my life already knew this, but it was news to me. Why are we always the last to know? Sigh.

I listened intently, took copious notes, and bought the book. I was all in.

The message God gave through Jan that day helped me move deeper into my becoming and literally changed my life. I have never been the same.

Pastor Peter Scazerro, author of *Emotionally Healthy Spirituality*, teaches that emotional health and spiritual maturity cannot be separated. One cannot be spiritually mature while remaining *emotionally immature*. How can I claim to be a grown-up Christian woman if my behaviors, reactions, and emotions are more reflective of a teenager? The answer is, I can't.

If you're wondering where you land as a mature Christian woman, here are some questions you can analyze:

- What is my initial response when I hear the word *no*?
- When conflict arises in one of my relationships, how do I handle it?
- Am I easily offended?
- Am I passive-aggressive?
- Do I control with anger or tantrums?
- Do I have a public self that is not in harmony with my private self?
- Am I applying God's truth to my life and seeing good fruit as I grow?
- Am I farther along in faith and trust than I was a year ago?

These are questions to ask ourselves when discerning how we're doing as growing Christian women—they are not meant to discourage or shame. Instead, we can examine ourselves with curiosity and grace, but also with an honest commitment that we can do better. We can use them to help us become.

Our maturity matters. Immature Christians can wreak havoc in the church. They confuse unbelieving family members and friends with behavior that does not match who they claim to be as Christ followers. In leadership positions, they can destroy the health of an organization, a church, or ministry team.

Living like a child in a woman's body is miserable, and it will directly affect your ability to move forward on the healing path.

Conversely, a mature Christian woman is a blessing to the body of Christ and to those in her sphere of influence. She resides in a place of discernment, patience, and wisdom. This woman gives grace freely and refuses to take part in little girl antics, including unhealthy ways of eating and taking care of her body. She is not easily duped or tempted.

A mature Christian woman doesn't beat her body into submission as if it needs to be conquered. Even if she'd like to improve it, she's finally learned to be comfortable in her own skin. She understands there is no perfection—only progress.

A mature Christ-follower knows if she is breathing, there is time to grow. The words "this is just how I am" never leave her mouth. She gives herself plenty of room for becoming.

Maturity is not a destination that magically comes with age. It is a place we can choose to live in at any time or circumstance, thanks to a good God who always gives us the ability to become our very best.

SOUL FITNESS: Strengthening Your Core

Looking over today's questions, what jumped out at you? In what ways might you reflect immaturity? Why do you think this is? Write one step you can take this week to grow up in this area—give yourself grace as you do. Write down the names of women in your life who display Christ-like maturity. Which of their attributes are examples to you?

PRAYER

Jesus, I am so tired of my childish behavior. I want to be a grown-up Christian woman, but parts of me are not there yet. Please help me remember you are with me and cheering me on. Remind me to give grace to myself as I walk this imperfect path of becoming. Send mature women to me as an encouragement and example. Thank you for always giving me the opportunity to grow. Amen.

DAY 12

*For I am the L*ORD *who heals you.*

Exodus 15:26 NLT

I'd yo-yo dieted for thirteen years when my husband, Pat, and I became engaged at age twenty-four. I distinctly remember waking up the next morning with the ring on my finger. Admiring the sparkling diamond and gold band, I said to myself, *I'm going to be happy now. The weight will come off and all will be well.* Pat loved me unconditionally. I truly believed his love for me would fix my issues, and I would never have to diet again. Nice thought, but that was fantasy thinking.

The truth is my marriage didn't change a thing.

I'm grateful for every single day of the thirty-nine years Pat and I have been together. Though not perfect, our relationship is a faithful, loving partnership with our Lord Jesus at the center. A strong Christian marriage is an enormous blessing, and I don't take it for granted. My husband and I have grown and matured together. I thank God for my sweet husband, but he couldn't fix me.

In the early years after our marriage, my food issues didn't go away as I'd hoped, so I heaped shame on myself. Expecting Pat to fix me only made things worse. He didn't understand my behavior any more than I did. After all, I had a wonderful husband and three beautiful children. What more could I ask for? Why couldn't I get my act together and lose the weight once and for all?

I lived like this until I realized a life-changing truth: *Only God can fix what He has created. Only God can redeem a life. Only God can restore me to the person I was created to be. My husband cannot correct any of that.*

Look at it this way: if the love of a good man is the answer to our body image, food issues, and other related strongholds, what is a single or divorced woman to do? Does she just exist as half a human, and suffer in bondage until a man comes to fix and complete her?

What is a widowed woman to do? Does her self-esteem and self-worth go to the grave with her husband? Does she have to hurry and get another man so she'll be okay?

Of course, you know the answer. The unconditional love of a good man models Jesus's love for us and makes for a joyful and meaningful life. Marriage is an incredible blessing, but it cannot and will not fix you.

What if you have a husband, but he isn't supportive? The answer is the same. God is the fixer of who He has made. There comes a point when we must unequivocally believe that we are who God says we are, no matter what.

This is not to be insensitive to those who struggle in difficult marriages. That is a hard and lonely road. Our faithful God will meet you there too. But if we place our hope for healing our self-image, brokenness, or our shame in a man or any other human, we are standing on sinking sand.

All men will disappoint. Some will leave. Some will check out but stay. And all men will eventually die. God is the only one who never leaves, never changes, and never dies. He is always, always faithful. And He is forever committed to our becoming.

I know I am being very direct with you, but I believe this into my bones. You are fixable, but you must take your pain to the Lord, Jehovah Rapha, the God who heals. When we look to external circumstances or relationships to repair us, we miss countless opportunities to know and experience the deep, tender, and stunning attribute of God's healing.

SOUL FITNESS: Strengthening Your Core

Have you relied on your husband, children, or other relationships to fix you? Have you been waiting for a certain relationship to materialize, hoping it will be the answer to your brokenness? Sweet sister, the only relationship that can fix you is the one with your Creator.

PRAYER

God, forgive me for placing my hope in people instead of you. It isn't fair to them, and it isn't good for me. Thank you for being my Jehovah Rapha, the God who heals me. Praise your name. Amen.

DAY 13

For you formed my inward parts;
you knitted me together in my mother's womb.
I praise you, for I am fearfully and wonderfully made.

Psalm 139:13–14 ESV

The world comes to a complete stop when our baby granddaughter comes to visit. Her birth ushered in such a sweet time of life—Pat and I adore being Evie's Nonie and Grandpap. One of the best parts is having the time to sit, observe, and listen, watching this new little person discover the world. Let me give you a few things I noticed right away when feeding Evie.

- When Evie is hungry, she lets you know. Immediately. We have no trouble hearing and responding to her hunger cues.
- When she is full, she's done. It is not possible to get her to take more milk or cereal.
- Though she's fed on a schedule, sometimes Evie is hungry again before her next meal. We don't tell her she shouldn't be hungry and make her wait until she's "supposed" to eat. We feed her.
- Most of the time, she drinks her full bottle, and sometimes she doesn't. Her hunger fluctuates.

Without outside voices drowning out her hunger and fullness cues, Evie could go on feeding her body this way for the rest of her life.

We were created to eat intuitively. Our very survival depends on this from the moment we are born. We drink when we are thirsty. We lie down when we are tired. If we ignore our thirst and rest cues, we will become sick, and endanger our health. Our hunger and fullness cues are the same. Why do we ignore them?

Here are only a few examples:

- As children, we were part of the "clean plate club." We couldn't leave the table unless we finished every bite—even when we reported we were full.

- Our diet-conscious mothers ignored their own bodies and taught us to do the same. "You can't be hungry—you had breakfast an hour ago. Drink some water or chew some gum until it's lunchtime."

- To survive diets, we ignored our hunger. If we were out of our allotted food for the day, we went to bed hungry. Then, we over-ate because we didn't fuel sooner or give our bodies enough. We ignored our fullness cues. It became a vicious cycle we couldn't get out of.

Your hunger cues may have become overridden, covered up, and silenced, but they are still trying to tell you what you need. Once you relearn to tune in to and trust your body, you will hear them again.

Once you start listening to your natural cues, some days you will only feel hungry at mealtimes. On other occasions, your stomach will feel empty an hour after breakfast. But this time, instead of shaming yourself, you will eat a healthy snack.

Your hunger will fluctuate. It's normal and part of being human.

As you learn, you will choose healthy food most of the time, because it makes you feel good and gives you consistent energy. It's okay to eat something just because it tastes good too.

You'll limit foods that make you feel sluggish or bloated. It's not because they're bad or forbidden, they just don't react well with your body.

Returning to how we were designed to interact with food is an imperfect journey, but it is one worth traveling. Expect trial and error as you become an expert on you. But, if you stick with it, you will relearn to be in sync with the body God gave you.

Sweet sister, feeding your body what it needs, when it needs it, translates into peace with food and peace within you. Can you imagine how free you will become? Let today be the day you begin trusting your body again.

SOUL FITNESS: Strengthening Your Core

Look at the hunger and fullness chart on page 131. As you relearn to trust your hunger and fullness cues, the goal is to eat and stop between the 3 to 7 range on the chart. Try it over the next few days, paying attention to how your body feels and what it is communicating to you. Record any observations with curiosity and grace. Remember, imperfection is expected as you rebuild trust with your body.

PRAYER

Heavenly Father, your Word tells me I am fearfully and wonderfully made. Please give me the patience and grace I need to reconnect with how you created me. Please help me honor my miraculous body as I become fully who you want me to be. Amen

DAY 14

But they soon forgot what he had done
and did not wait for his plan to unfold.

Psalm 106:13

The book of Exodus in the Bible provides the details of a miraculous story of liberation—but this historical account has its share of issues. Even after God miraculously brought the Israelites out of captivity and provided for them in the wilderness, His people, the ones He rescued, never stepped foot in the Promised Land. Why? Their forgetfulness led to unbelief.

In dramatic fashion, Almighty God swept in, pulled the Israelite people out of generations of slavery, and provided for them in the desert wilderness. He promised a beautiful, spacious place to live in freedom. And after all that, they forgot what He'd done and fell into unbelief. This original generation wandered in the desert until the last person died. Only the next generation saw the Promised Land. This leads me to wonder.

How do you forget your God parted the Red Sea? How do you forget manna raining down from heaven to feed you day by day? How do you forget the ways the Lord protected your family from enemies and provided for all your needs? How on earth do you forget the miracles?

Every time I encounter the passage about the Israelites' journey to freedom, it's like having a mirror held up to my face. I am forced to reflect on seasons where I waited for God to answer my cries, then all too quickly, I failed to recall His past provision and care. My forgetfulness led to periods of unbelief.

Unbelief not only comes in the form of denying God's existence. Unbelief can show up in the life of a Christian when we are forgetful about God's provision and wonder if He will really come through for us again.

If we apply this to our healing journey, there are similarities. Food restriction provides false security when it is truly captivity. Dieting can feel like we're wandering in a desert too. When we search the horizon, we can't see the Promised Land yet. We fear it will never appear and are tempted to turn back. We doubt if the Promised Land even exists.

Resolve is most important in these moments. When waiting seems endless, and our faith is wavering, we need to *remember*.

Recalling the ways the Lord has led, protected, and provided for us is critical. At the front of our minds, we must keep a record of all the times He's come through for us over our lifetime. Doubt has a hard time dominating your brain when it's busy remembering how God has cared for you in the past.

In Joshua 4, God performed yet another miracle for the people of Israel. This generation entered the Promised Land, but only after navigating the Jordan River that blocked their way. Just as He did a generation before at the Red Sea, God parted the waters for the people to cross. When they arrived on the other side, God, through Joshua, commanded some men to go back to the middle of the river, collect twelve stones, and bring them back to the camp. He then instructed them to create a memorial with the stones to remind future generations of God's faithfulness to His people. He knew they'd forget and would need a reminder.

It makes sense that God knew stones from the *middle* of the journey across the Jordan would carry a particular meaning. In the millennia since, human nature has not changed. We all need reminders to keep going even when we can't see the destination. God is the One who will get you safely to the other side.

The middle part of any journey to freedom is the most stressful. Travelers become weary at this juncture. The road feels long, and the grumbling begins. They think of turning back, wondering if the attempt is futile. Many never make it to the Promised Land.

We become emboldened and strong when we remember Jehovah Jireh, meaning the God who provides. Just as He provided for us yesterday (remember?), He will also provide today and tomorrow. Lay your doubt aside and resolve to arrive in the Promised Land. Your attempts are not futile—keep going. You can confidently move forward into the spacious place of freedom He has been waiting for you. Each step you take is part of your becoming.

SOUL FITNESS: Strengthening Your Core

Recall all the ways God provided for you in the past. Make a list or timeline of when He came through for you over your lifetime. If you are struggling with unbelief, where does it come from? How does remembering God's previous provision help you with your unbelief today?

PRAYER

Lord, Jehovah Jireh, you are the God who provides. You know what I need even before I ask. You have provided for me spiritually, emotionally, and physically all throughout my life. Thank you from the bottom of my heart. When unbelief seeps in, help me remember your goodness to me. Amen.

DAY 15

God does not view things the way people do. People look
on the outward appearance, but the LORD looks at the heart.

1 Samuel 16:7 NET

We've all seen them. The diet culture is infamous for posting before and after pictures. As I've learned more and more about the mindset of a woman who struggles with weight and body image, I now understand these images don't even begin to tell the whole story. Real life is so much more complicated.

One person's before is another person's now, and for every person feeling inspired, there's an equal number of others feeling shame. The truth about weight loss before and after pictures is they're hurtful, and in truth, don't tell you much of anything. I am not saying some aren't motivated or inspired by them, but is what they are longing for true?

Images like these simply show a person's outward appearance at two specific moments in time. But what about the rest of her story?

Here's just some of what is left out:

- What did she do to lose the weight? Starve, skip meals, overexercise?

- Has she kept the weight off? If so, is she using extreme measures to stay there?

- Is she still obsessed and in bondage to counting numbers, rigid record keeping, restrictive eating, and the whims of the scale?
- Is her body healthy? Is her mind?

Just think of celebrities who become spokespeople for famous dieting programs. We see their dramatic before and after pictures and wish we could experience the same transformation. And yet, with all their resources, they typically gain it all back. The media brings out those before and after pictures again, this time, publicly shaming the celebrity.

A minute ago, they were experts on losing weight—the epitome of health and beauty. Now they are a failure. It isn't until they lose the weight again that they fall back into the good graces of the public—for a time. Then the cycle continues.

We truly live in a culture where our value consists of youth, beauty, and thin bodies, no matter what it takes to get or stay there. Before and after pictures keep the focus on outward appearance above all else, rather than true health and well-being. Thank goodness we don't have to live this way.

Our God changes us from the inside out. He looks at our heart. He reaches into the places that truly need redeeming and sets us free.

- There are no after pictures of a woman whose inner life has been completely transformed.

- There are no after pictures of a woman whose health issues are now under control after treating her body well.

- There are no after pictures of a woman who no longer treats her body as her sworn enemy.

- There are no after pictures of a woman who is finally at peace, treating her body with grace and care, reconnected to her hunger cues. Someone who has eliminated the shame from her life.

The measurements of "after" require us to document or prove our results to others. But we do not need to use outdated and shame-inducing measurements to tell us if we are free or not.

John 8:36 tells us, "So if the Son sets you free, you will be free indeed." The original Hebrew word for *indeed* in this passage means "really, truly, and actually." This means Jesus will actually, really, and truly heal us! Isn't that all we need to know?

A woman who has done the very different-than-dieting hard work of allowing God to heal her knows the night and day difference of her *real* before and after. She understands her becoming cannot be captured in a photo or on a scale. Her transformation is between her and the Healer. They both know what was and what now is, and truly, that is all that matters.

SOUL FITNESS: Strengthening Your Core

You can see shame as the thread that weaves its way through every part of our issues with food and body image. Have you ever considered how before and after pictures contribute to the problem? What other features of the diet culture cultivate shame? How have they affected you? Journal your thoughts on what really matters as you continue on your healing path.

PRAYER

God, it's amazing to think you will actually, really, truly set me free! I am so thankful you are most concerned with my heart and healing my hurting soul. Thank you for opening my eyes to the many ways shame has crept into my life and helping me become your truth of me. I am praising you with each step toward freedom. Amen.

DAY 16

She is clothed with strength and dignity,
and she laughs without fear of the future.

Proverbs 31:25 NLT

Let's think about growing older. I noticed the first dreaded signs of aging when I was in my early thirties, at least that's what I thought they were. I was all dressed up for a Christmas party, wearing a beautiful black velvet dress. My hair was in an updo with a pearl and rhinestone comb holding it all together. I felt pretty that night, until I took a fateful trip to the ladies' room.

While washing my hands at the sink, I looked up at the mirror and my heart sank. Despite the velvet and pearls, all I saw were wrinkles around my eyes. It totally shocked me. They jumped out at me as if they were under a magnifying glass. I thought to myself, *As if fighting with my body isn't miserable enough, now I have to worry about wrinkles.*

I returned to the party, not feeling pretty anymore.

Looking back now, I realize how silly I was. I had three small children at home, and I was probably just a tired mama. But it's not uncommon for women—young or old—to fear their changing bodies.

Society's message is loud and clear: aging is bad—do everything you can to fight against it. Even though increasingly younger women fret about wrinkles, women have been seeking anti-aging remedies for centuries.

There is nothing wrong with wanting to look your best and to soften the effects of age. It is *what we tell ourselves* and what we falsely believe that creates problems.

Whether we are young, old, or in between, our body image issues are actually not about size or aging. The real stronghold root originates with the stories we tell ourselves about our bodies and the belief that what we look like determines our worth. This is why it is so important to allow God's Word to reframe the whole picture of who we are.

I am sixty-four years old. My friends will tell you I've gone into "older woman status" kicking and screaming. My resistance isn't only about age marching across my face; it's also about the realization that (as my husband says) we only have a little runway left. I still have so much I want to learn and do.

However, once I accepted my situation and thought it through, I landed on the importance of my higher priorities.

- I do not want to spend the rest of my years in bondage to a food/dieting/body image mess.
- I want to be free.
- I want to be as mentally, spiritually, and physically healthy as possible.
- I need to be fully present in the life of my friends and family.
- I want to keep up with my grandchildren.
- My dream is to be a fully mature Christian woman serving Jesus and His church until the day I die.

I realized I couldn't be any of those things if I continued to wrestle with The Shamer over who or what I believed. And so, I stopped struggling. I quit wasting any more of my precious and fleeting time on pointless concerns, fears, worries, or shame.

The woman described in Proverbs 31 "laughs without fear of the future." She is not afraid of the season that is coming. She doesn't cling to something that is ending. This sister lives in reality and embraces the life God has given her. Without worry!

Our bodies were created to change. We are not supposed to look like we did ten or twenty years ago. Most of us will never fit back into our wedding dress or get down to what we weighed as a teenager. Seriously, in the scheme of things, nothing of vanity is important.

What *is* important is becoming the healthiest, strongest version of you, both inside and out. It's important to get on with your fleeting life. It's important to let God set you free. The runway is getting shorter—there is no more time to waste.

SOUL FITNESS: Strengthening Your Core

Whether you are twenty or eighty, I want you to ponder and journal the blessings of the age you are today. Write what you love and appreciate about your body and how it has served you over the years. Then, thinking about your future, record what concerns you and what you are excited about. If there is anything you need to leave behind that is keeping you from getting on with your life, write it down. Ask God to help you let it go, so you can become the best version of you.

PRAYER

Dear Father, thank you for my life. Thank you for the years you have given me. I want to steward them well and not chase futile dreams. I want my dreams for me to match yours. Help me age gracefully no matter what season I am in now. Help me let go of anything that is in the way of my becoming your best for me. Amen.

DAY 17

"Be still, and know that I am God."

Psalm 46:10 ESV

Most writers and speakers understand it is important to know your audience. It's dangerous to assume you already know what they're thinking or feeling. Even though I'm a woman who's struggled with body image and food for decades, I understood the value of gathering insights for this book through an anonymous survey. I sent out a simple four-question poll with multiple choice answers. As always, I found women eager to help—their responses were truly insightful and a little surprising.

When asked to name the obstacle between where they are today and their wellness goals, most women reported they were "lazy and lacked willpower." Since this was a multiple-choice question, they could have chosen an answer that did not point the finger toward themselves, but woman after woman did. My heart sank when I read the responses.

Sister, laziness and willpower are not your problem. That's the shame talking once again.

A woman who's been on diets for decades, restricting her calories to nothing, resisting cake on her own birthday, and eating food she doesn't even like, does not lack willpower. She has it in spades.

A woman who plots and plans every bite she's going to put in her mouth is not lazy. If she cooks two dinners a day, every day, one for her family and one for herself, she isn't lazy. And she certainly doesn't lack discipline.

Obviously, a woman who loses weight, gains it all back but keeps trying repeatedly to re-lose and keep it off, isn't short on will or power.

When we believe paralyzing lies that tell us we are lazy and lack will-power, we've got it wrong. God never asks us to strive, strain, and struggle our way through life. Striving, straining, and struggling is trying to be good, trying to be strong, trying to control. We keep trying, trying, trying, when God simply asks us to surrender.

Psalm 46:10, our verse of the day, is familiar to most of us. We stitch it on pillows and hang it on our walls, but do we understand the full meaning?

The Hebrew word for "be still" is *raphah*, defined as: "to release, let go, desist, or cease your efforts."

Here are a few more translations of the verse:

- "Stop striving and know that I am God" (NASB).
- "Stop your fighting—and know that I am God" (HCSB).
- "Be at peace in the knowledge that I am God" (BBE).
- "Let go [of your concerns]! Then you will know that I am God" (GW).

I find comfort in the small inflections that sharpen my perspective of God's meaning. Though each biblical translation tweaks the exact wording just a bit, the core meaning does not change. The variances simply help me see more clearly.

Every translation of Psalm 46:10 says we are safe to place our struggles into God's hands because we know Him. You can't trust someone you don't know. To know God is to understand His character and acknowledge His sovereignty over your life. We learn who He is through His living Word.

Psalm 46:10 reminds us that surrender does not always mean giving up or throwing in the towel. We humans often surrender as a last resort, but like so many things we resist doing that are good for us, stepping beyond the bondage of food and body obsessions is something we'll wish we had done sooner. We cannot become free if we do not first become still so God can do His work in us.

The real obstacle between you and your healing is not willpower or laziness. Attempts to recover under your own power is the issue in your way. Let's clear the path by becoming still today.

SOUL FITNESS: Strengthening Your Core

Read Exodus 14:14, Psalm 37:7, and Psalm 62:5. Look up various translations of the verses to broaden your understanding of God's meaning. How do these passages, along with Psalm 46:10, impact your thoughts on relying on God's power and not your own? Write down a statement describing what "release, let go, desist, or cease your efforts" looks like for you.

PRAYER

Jesus, I admit I have been trying to find healing through my power and not yours. It is all too much for me, but it's not too much for you. Today, I am turning my struggles with my body over to your capable hands. I surrender. Thank you for being the One who always fights for me and gives me rest from striving in this world. Amen.

DAY 18

Instead, we will speak the truth in love, growing in every way more and more like Christ, who is the head of his body, the church.

Ephesians 4:15 NLT

Since many of us who struggle with food and body image strongholds have the disease to please, we may not speak up for ourselves or others when it's time to do so. We worry we won't be accepted, or that we will be perceived as mean or angry if we tell the truth. We don't want to disrupt peace, however fragile it may be. What if we are exposed and rejected? This concern is yet another consequence of stuffing our emotions and dimming our light. I know this too well.

My mom often told a story about me when I was in the third grade. Until then, I'd had a happy, nurturing experience in elementary school, but at eight years old, I was placed in a class with a cold and unkind teacher. She was stern, used sharp words, and exhibited little compassion toward the children in her class.

Back then, we learned our times tables in the third grade. Every day after returning to class from lunch, the teacher would drill us individually in front of the class. If you were successful, you got a sticker on a chart by her desk. If you messed up, a mean-spirited comment followed. She mistakenly believed that shame was an effective motivator, but it had the opposite effect on me.

Fearing her anger, I routinely froze when it was my turn to recite my times tables. If I hesitated or answered wrong, she humiliated me, questioning whether I was lying about practicing at home, and sent me back to my seat. This awful scenario was repeated daily.

When I came home for lunch each day, I begged my mother not to take me back to school. I cried and pleaded with her to let me stay home. After a few days of this, she became concerned. She arranged a meeting with the teacher to discuss how I was feeling.

Mom explained how frightened I was of her and related my daily lunch requests to stay home. To my mother's surprise, the teacher laughed and responded, "I can't believe she is crying and carrying on like that. No matter what I *do* or *say* to Laura, she never cries."

The result of that meeting ended not as I hoped. I was left in that classroom for the rest of the year. My parents felt I needed to learn to get along with difficult people. Sadly, that didn't happen. Although the teacher backed off, I still felt I had to lie low and stay quiet to survive.

A few years ago, when God was teaching me to stop stuffing my feelings, this long forgotten story came to mind. It was one of those aha moments when I realized I'd been conditioned to stuff and stay silent to get along.

Today, I'm different. I've become a woman who understands I am not dependent on anyone to speak up for me. You aren't either.

We are operating in God's truth when we advocate and insist on others treating us with respect and care. We should release the fear that we will be exposed and rejected if we speak up. Someone else's response to our words is not up to us, but speaking the truth when called for *is* our responsibility. When sharing hard truths, we must speak in love and listen to the Holy Spirit as He guides us. This is how we keep our heart in check.

Remember, the Lord always goes before you. He always has your back. And He will forever advocate on your behalf. Jesus will tend to you and contend for you. Friend, you have all you need to stand strong.

SOUL FITNESS: Strengthening Your Core

Float back in your mind to the earliest memory when you needed an adult to speak up for you. Write about the experience and the positive or negative impact it had on you. As an adult, how comfortable are you advocating for yourself in a way that honors you, others, and God?

PRAYER

God, I am often more interested in pleasing people than pleasing you. I need help to speak up for myself and for others in a way that is honoring to all. Please cure me of the disease to please. Help me become strong and true. Amen.

DAY 19

Do not gloat over me, my enemy!
Though I have fallen, I will rise.
Though I sit in darkness,
the Lord will be my light.

Micah 7:8

What has living in bondage cost you? What parts of your life did you miss out on because of your struggles with body image and food? How has your struggle impacted those closest to you?

Have you ever:

- Turned down social invitations from friends after calculating you gained weight since the last time they saw you?

- Avoided getting in the pool with your kids because you did not want to be seen in a bathing suit?

- Held back on intimacy with your husband, even though he loves you as you are?

- Not been fully present at family celebrations because you could not stop thinking about food and worrying that people were judging what you put on your plate?

- Missed out on the joy of anticipating an important milestone (weddings, graduations, reunions, etc.) because you were consumed with how skinny you could get before the big day?
- Passed on your toxic thinking about food and body image to your children?

I know it's a cringe-worthy list. I've struggled with many, plus a few more. Let me point out the insidiousness of shame once again.

Although it may feel counter-intuitive, counting the cost of our bondage is another key to freedom. Please don't fear the process. Being honest with yourself is critical to your healing. And if you think captivity to food and body image hasn't cost you anything, think again.

Our God, who is compassionate and kind, calls us out of the shadows and into the light where truth lives. Once we come clean and admit the diet culture has cost us way more than the money we've thrown away on it, we take a major step forward. And God understands. It's safe to be our true selves in His presence. He knows everything about us anyway.

Scripture tells us that Jesus is full of grace and truth. Notice the order of the two words. Grace always precedes truth when describing His characteristics. They work in tandem. He does not possess 50 percent grace and 50 percent truth. He is full of both. As His wayward children, we need it all.

The fourth step in the Alcoholics Anonymous twelve-step program is to take a fearless personal inventory of oneself. In the program's words, we "made a searching and fearless moral inventory of ourselves." This crucial task is considered the foundational step for lasting recovery. It is also one of the hardest for people to complete.

Taking a searching personal inventory is a crucial task that applies to us too. And when we contemplate ourselves through in-depth, honest analysis, Satan always hurls the fiery dart of fear. He tells us that doing so will make us fall apart like Humpty Dumpty, never to be put back together again. That's just another one of his lies. Alcoholics Anonymous and other recovery programs have discovered taking a personal inventory and counting the cost puts us back together—it does not break us apart.

When you bravely count the cost of your bondage to food and body image, there is no question you will feel sorrow and repentance. That's a good thing. You may even need to have a courageous conversation or two. But, thanks to the healing power of God, once you take this action, you will experience relief and a lightness no weight loss plan can ever deliver.

The deeper you go into self-discovery, the more you will fully comprehend all God has restored in you. Fear and shame will be replaced with joy and gratitude. The significance and miracle of your recovery can only be understood through the lens of God's glorious grace and unvarnished truth.

Dear one, you've had a hard time. The enemy has plotted to keep you in darkness and despair. Today, let's silence his mocking voice and bring all he has tried to keep hidden into the light. Let's become bravely honest and let God set us free.

SOUL FITNESS: Strengthening Your Core

Make a list of what bondage has cost you. Sit with God while you ask Him to bring truth to your mind. Be present in His grace. Feel your feelings. Grieve the losses. Receive His love and compassion for you. Write the word *grace* next to each "cost." His grace covers all the truth He will reveal to you. Don't wait another minute—start becoming free today. Praise His name.

PRAYER

Heavenly Father, I have felt afraid to face the reality of my bondage. I would prefer to believe it has only affected me, but now I understand it has affected others too. Please forgive me. I want to live in the light with you. Thank you for covering me with your grace and speaking to me with truth. Amen.

NOURISHMENT FOR YOUR SOUL

I do not at all understand the mystery of grace—only that it meets us where we are but does not leave us where it found us.

Anne Lamott

DAY 20

*The Lord God said, "It is not good for the man to be alone.
I will make a helper suitable for him."*

Genesis 2:18

It all went off the rails in the garden. In the first book of the Bible, Eve made a fateful decision that changed everything. Eve listened to the wrong voice and Adam listened to Eve. Both forgot *who* they were and *Whose* they were. Because of this chain of events, our perfect creation was shattered, and the world was set on a course that led directly to the cross. From that moment forward, God began His plan of restoration. Humankind needed a Savior to turn everything right side up again.

With all kinds of "wrong voices" around us, we can forget who we are and Whose we are too. When we take our eyes off the Creator, as Adam and Eve did, and listen to what's whispered (or sometimes shouted) in our ears, we buy into the great lie. In some form or another, we're told, "God didn't mean what He said."

So today, let's be very clear on what God says about us as His female creation and about our unique role as women in this world.

In Genesis 1 and 2, the Bible says God created the heavens and the earth. As He completed each part, He declared everything was good—until something wasn't. It was not good for man to be alone. He needed a "helper," and so God created woman.

When I was a young girl, the word *helper* didn't sound particularly inspiring to me. Some translations use the term "help meet," which only made my dislike worse. Because of incorrect teaching on the subject, I believed that a woman's main role was to simply help her husband. But there's a problem with that philosophy.

If we were created only to be helpers to husbands, what does a single woman do? What is her purpose? Does she only get to live out a partial life and calling? What about widows or women who have been left by their husbands? Is there no value for them?

The English word "helper" in Genesis 2:18 is translated from the Hebrew word "Ezer." This beautiful name is one God uses to name Himself throughout the Old Testament, but in this one instance, He refers to the woman as Ezer too. It is mostly used as a *military term* and translated means "rescue, strength, and power."

These attributes, which Scripture upholds, define woman as a warrior. And why not? We make up more than half of the church. Even though it is not God's primary desire, the fact is that women are often the spiritual leaders of their families. When people are asked who led them to Christ, their answer is more often than not a mother, grandmother, or aunt. Never get in the way of a praying woman!

As women, we have big hearts that long for justice. We will fight passionately for our friends, family, and important causes. Like Mary, the mother of Jesus, we are strong women—from birth to death.

Of course, this doesn't mean we are powerful in our own strength. All our attributes begin and end with God. It is His power and might that fuel an Ezer.

Yes, if we are married, we serve and help our husbands as they help and serve us. But there is so much more to the role God has given to us women, whether we are single, married, widowed, or divorced.

There is no doubt our culture, with all its deceptions, has tried to shatter God's intended image of women. Please don't listen to the lying voices. We have God's Word to define us. He doesn't mince words. He doesn't hide the truth. His design and plan cannot be redefined. Stand firm in who you are and Whose you are. You are a warrior who belongs to God.

This world was not complete until a woman's rescuing, strong, and powerful presence entered the scene. Females were not an afterthought or an add-on. Eve was the crowning glory of creation. God knew this world needed our distinctly feminine presence, and together with man, through us He revealed His full image to the world. Don't let anyone tell you otherwise.

SOUL FITNESS: Strengthening Your Core

Satan has remained committed to distorting the female image since he met Eve in the garden. It's important for us to have a clear and right understanding of who we are as God's distinctly female creation. Journal your thoughts on why this is important for you in your day-to-day life. Consider ways that you are or long to be an Ezer. How does knowing you are the crowning glory of creation impact your relationship with your body, mind, and soul?

PRAYER

Thank you, God, for naming me Ezer, a name you call yourself. Thank you for creating me as a warrior. Please protect me from the enemy's lies that tell me I am less than or not enough. Help me become confident in who I am as a co-bearer of your image. Please use me to reflect your specific design for women into a very lost and confused world. Amen.

DAY 21

And I'll stride freely through wide open spaces
as I look for your truth and your wisdom;
Then I'll tell the world what I find,
speak out boldly in public, unembarrassed.

Psalm 119:45–46 MSG

One principle of healing from *anything* is reclaiming your voice. One of the steps to recovery is allowing the real you to come forward to be seen and heard.

Some females are chatty, excitable, and emotional. Others are quiet, pensive, and ponder more than they speak. There is no right or wrong way to be a woman, contrary to the lies we may have been sold. In a culture that supposedly celebrates authenticity, there are plenty of mixed messages coming our way:

- Be yourself, but tone it down.
- Be yourself, but rein it in.
- Be yourself, but be more assertive.
- Be yourself, but . . .

Even though I grew up in the middle of the 1960s women's movement, I was taught that if I attended a meeting with men at work, church, or anywhere else, the best practice was to not speak like a woman. I was advised that men like short conversations, few words, and no emotion. If I wanted to be taken seriously, I had to somehow silence the feminine part of me when I added my voice to the mix.

Decades later, of course, I believe it's essential to bring our full feminine selves to the conversation. After all, this is authentically who we are, and our uniquely female perspective is needed. Without it, there can be no full picture.

Jesus, our Creator, understood this, even in a culture that viewed women as property. Their testimonies were widely considered wholly unreliable. In Jesus's day, feminine voices were silenced—but He wouldn't stand for it.

He did not condemn women who dared to use their voices. In fact, He empowered them to speak and act at critical moments in His ministry.

- Women bore witness to the crucifixion and were the first at the resurrection.
- Jesus's ministry was financially supported by women.
- He entrusted a woman with the truth when He told Martha, "I am the resurrection, and the life."
- Jesus inspired a Samaritan woman to use her voice to tell everyone in her town about Him when He met her at the well.
- When Mary of Bethany sat at His feet to soak up His teaching, her sister asked Jesus to put her back in the kitchen where she belonged. But Jesus said she had chosen the better thing.
- Women were among Christ's disciples.

The sum of Jesus's interaction with women is this: we have a place at any table, and it is imperative that we show up as our true selves.

Friend, shame tells us we must contort every part of us into something different from who we are. It isn't just what we weigh, what we eat, or whether we think we are pretty enough. Shame tells us all of our being is wrong, every single bit, so you might as well fade into the background and quiet down.

Don't you do it. Jesus called women out of the shadows and restored them just as He found them—bleeding, broken, mentally ill, sinful, and desperate. *He received them when their full emotions were on display.* They didn't have to tone themselves down or dial it back for Him to take them seriously. He doesn't expect you to either.

You may feel you're invisible and pushed to the side, but that isn't how Jesus sees you. He is extending His hand to pull you out of the shadows, where shame has placed you. He wants you to become more of your God-designed self, not less.

Come forward and add your authentic voice and feminine self to the conversation. Come as you are. Without you, we are all missing your unique perspective, experiences, and personality. The world needs you to become—whether it realizes it or not.

SOUL FITNESS: Strengthening Your Core

How comfortable are you showing up as your authentic self? Have you picked up messages that tell you it's best to stay small and out of the way? What is your reaction to knowing Jesus received women with their full emotions on display?

PRAYER

Father, through Jesus's interactions with women, you encourage your daughters to become our true feminine selves. Thank you for always valuing who we are and what we bring to the table. May we honor you in all the places you send us, bringing glory to your name. Amen.

DAY 22

Those who look to him are radiant;
their faces are never covered with shame.

Psalm 34:5

You're kind of pretty for a fat girl," a boy said to me in English class when I was thirteen years old. This is but one of the many back-handed compliments spoken to me over the years. I could make a long list—I am sure you can too.

The "beauty bar" set for women in our culture is impossible to reach. I don't know who made the rules, but I found that no sooner did I contort myself into an attribute deemed as beautiful and acceptable, the bar moved, and I had to jump even higher. I could starve myself into a skinny body, but couldn't change my round face, turned-up nose, or short legs. I still have them all. LOL.

Today, we have injections, fillers, implants, and surgery to alter what dieting can't. We inject things in and suck things out in hopes of achieving an acceptable body. We use filters before posting any photos of ourselves on social media. Add an aging and changing body to the situation, and we're left with three choices:

- Keep futilely chasing the elusive standard of beauty set forth by our culture.

- Throw in the towel, declare yourself hopeless, and hide your body away.

- Reject the game, choose to believe what God says about beauty, and liberate yourself from the craziness.

I am here to tell you: for Christian women, the third choice is the only choice. In God's economy, *beautiful* has a completely different definition.

Yes, we want to look our best. Yes, we are free to take very good care of our bodies, and that includes our outward appearance. Yes, many of us enjoy cute outfits, makeup, jewelry, and feeling pretty. But some women don't, and that is okay.

From the time I was born, my grandmother said to me, "Pretty is as pretty does." I remember her words to this day and pray them over my infant granddaughter. One day, when she is older, I will speak them to her too. I will say, "Evie, a beautiful girl has a beautiful heart. Pretty is as pretty does."

I know that may sound trite, but it's true. Think of it like this: when you name the beautiful women in your life, some may not measure high on the "pretty" scale by the world's standards. What beautiful women do possess is a warm, inviting, forgiving, empathetic, kind, and humble soul. A beautiful woman is comfortable as her true self and the people around her feel safe to be their true selves too. Breathe in these life-giving words:

> She was beautiful, but not like those girls in magazines. She was beautiful, for the way she thought. She was beautiful, for the sparkle in her eyes when she talked about something she loved. She was beautiful, for her ability to make other people smile, even if she was sad. No, she wasn't beautiful for something as temporary as her looks. She was beautiful, deep down to her soul. She is beautiful. (Source Unknown)

A beautiful girl has a beautiful heart. A woman who is becoming understands that pretty is as pretty does.

SOUL FITNESS: Strengthening Your Core

Oh sister, this may be a hard one, but I want you to record all the ways you are beautiful on the inside. Don't skip over this. Record all the lovely attributes of beautiful you.

PRAYER

Lord, as a woman, I find it hard to deal with the world's idea of beauty. Help me to see myself the way you see me. Help me to define beauty through your eyes. Help me to become truly beautiful in a way that sparkles from my soul to my skin. Amen.

Still Becoming

DAY 23

See, I have written your name on the palms of my hands.

Isaiah 49:16 NLT

Our son Matthew is the youngest of our three boys. I honestly don't know how or when it all started, but one of his two older brothers began calling him "Cashew." The name stuck, and for the first two years of Matthew's life, he was called Cashew at home. Even now, twenty-eight years later, my husband gives Matthew a can of cashews on his birthday. It's a silly inside family joke.

You know how it goes, a name appears, and the family goes with it. Sometimes, it sticks for a lifetime.

One Sunday morning when Matthew was two, we were at church. He played in the nursery while Pat and I were in the service. After church was over, we headed down the hall to pick him up, but when we arrived at the nursery door, Matthew wasn't in the room. The nursery attendants were mortified to realize he had slipped out the door! The hallway was packed with Sunday school parents picking up their kids. We immediately started looking for him within the sea of people.

Suddenly, a man we'd never met before appeared in the hallway holding Matthew. He walked toward us, calling out to the crowd, "Whose baby is this? I found him in the parking lot, standing behind a truck. He says his name is Cashew!"

I'm sure I don't have to tell you how grateful we were to this brother in Christ for rescuing our son. With church letting out, we shuddered to think of what could have happened, if he hadn't come along.

After all the anxiety calmed down, we had a good laugh over Matthew telling the man his name was Cashew. We had no idea he didn't know his real name. After that, we made sure he understood his true moniker. It's important to know your proper name.

Have you been called by something that is not your real name? Like Matthew, you may have heard the name so often it replaced the one you were given at birth. Sometimes, the name sticks for a lifetime.

I had picked up several over the years. Mine were fat, ugly, stupid, damaged, and lazy. There were others too. Tragically, these paralyzing labels took root and defined me until I learned to replace them with the truth from God's Word.

My sister, if you have names that are hurtful to your soul, let's replace them with what your Father calls you. You were named by the One who chose you long before your appearance in your mother's womb. These true names don't change, no matter your experiences, your heartaches, or your failures.

According to Scripture, your Father calls you:

- Forgiven (Isaiah 43:25)
- Daughter (2 Corinthians 6:18)
- Beautiful (Isaiah 62:3)
- Chosen (1 Peter 2:9)
- Loved (Isaiah 43:4)
- Free (Jeremiah 29:12–14a)
- Blessed (Luke 1:45)
- Mine (Isaiah 43:1)

God has written your true name in the palm of His hand, and you can rest assured it encompasses the list above. You are treasured and loved. Let the names *He calls you* define you. Allow them to take root in your heart and soul. Become who God says you are.

SOUL FITNESS: Strengthening Your Core

Look up the Scriptures beside each one of your God-given names. Which ones mean the most regarding your current struggles with body image and disordered eating? Why?

PRAYER

God, please bring your names for me to mind as I go about my days. When old recordings want to play in my head, please help me replace those lies with the truth of what you call me. Thank you for writing my name on the palm of your hand. Amen.

DAY 24

A cheerful heart is good medicine.

Proverbs 17:22

I've eliminated the word *exercise* from my vocabulary. I know words are just words, but this change has helped me reframe my thinking on the subject. I like the term *joyful movement.* You can call it whatever you like.

My dad, who was an avid runner, used to tell me that if I didn't run five times a week for at least thirty minutes each day, I might as well not do it at all. He meant well, but this played right into my type-A, perfectionist personality. The apple (me) didn't fall far from his tree.

Dad's admonishment messed with my black-and-white, all-or-nothing thinking. In my estimation, perfection was always the goal, and anything else wasn't worth the effort. If I didn't see flawless results in the timespan I wanted, I didn't bother. Sadly, I have a long history of signing up for all kinds of fitness programs without completing them. Yes, I confess I'm an exercise-class dropout.

Movement benefits us beyond helping us lose weight. It relieves anxiety, clears our minds, gives us energy, and lifts our spirits. Taking a brisk walk on a spring morning or a fall evening helps us mentally, spiritually, and emotionally, while it pumps our hearts and firms our muscles.

I've discovered if I take a walk whenever I feel anxious, the stress lifts and I return home in a much better mood. Walking alone gives us time to pray, think, and ponder. A walk with a friend offers us a sweet time to chat, and as we women do, to try and solve all the world's problems. A stroll with your husband provides a way to connect and share joy together.

There is room for many types of movement in your life when you take nothing off the table. Choose what works for you. Be flexible enough to change your activities with the earth's seasons and your stage of life. What we want to get away from is the legalism, obsession, and perfectionism that often comes with rigidity. Life is too short for unreasonable expectations.

Most of us already understand that moving our bodies is a vital part of health and wholeness, but it is also a key component to recovering from food and body image strongholds. Joyful movement helps us connect with our bodies. How the movement makes you feel mentally, emotionally, physically, and spiritually will fine-tune your ability to listen to what your body is saying to you.

Noticing and listening to these connections will lead you to a balanced life. What a blessed relief following your natural rhythms offers, after living with disorder for so long. But remember—this isn't an all-or-nothing proposition. There is no right or wrong way to move, but I can tell you from experience, this anti-exercise, recovering perfectionist girl finally understands the connection between my comprehensive healing and motion.

Legalism tells you exercise is the price you must pay to make up for cheating on your diet. This leads to the black-and-white thinking that can fuel an obsession with exercise or the shame of giving up. One may think a fixation with exercise is better than a food compulsion, but your God wants more than that for you. He wants you to become totally free.

Legalism leaves no space for those who have physical limitations. The flip side is grace, where there is space for everyone.

So, come as you are. Come as you can. Moving your body joyfully is a vital part of learning to hear its voice and to treat it with respect and honor. Part of becoming is learning to listen and taking action.

SOUL FITNESS: Strengthening Your Core

What are your favorite ways to move your body? What are the joyful aspects of moving in this way? What are the benefits to your physical, mental, emotional, and spiritual health? How do you feel after your body has experienced this kind of motion?

PRAYER

Jesus, I come before you today with gratitude for my body. I want to move it joyfully, treating it with respect and honor. I am sorry for the times I treated myself poorly. Help me become more in tune to the connection between my body, mind, and spirit. Amen.

DAY 25

He brought me out into a spacious place;
he rescued me because he delighted in me.

2 Samuel 22:20

I know I'm dating myself, but travel back to 1965 with me. *The Sound of Music*, a movie starring Julie Andrews, was released to a public still reeling from the assassination of John F. Kennedy. By November 1966, *The Sound of Music* had become the highest grossing film of all time. The music, written by Rogers and Hammerstein, remains one of the most successful soundtrack albums in history. When I was growing up, we knew all the songs by heart.

The opening scene of the movie is set in a lush, wide-open field at the top of an Austrian hillside, with majestic snow-topped peaks in the background. Julie Andrews appears. She is running toward us through the vast, green field. Her arms are open, she is joyfully singing, and her body is *twirling*.

All at once, the viewer is transported to that Austrian hilltop and can almost breathe in the clear crystal air, expansive space, sheer beauty of the setting, and Julie's uninhibited, contagious joy. We want to twirl on that hill with her.

I have a picture of myself taken on Easter Sunday when I was five years old. I am wearing the typical little girl Easter Sunday uniform of the era. A white dress with pink smocking, frilly lace socks that turn down at the ankles, patent leather Mary Jane shoes, and an Easter bonnet symbolized the moment.

I'm twirling in the photo. In fact, I'm spinning so fast that my dress is blurred, and my bonnet is missing. I imagine I felt so happy in my pretty clothes, so thrilled it was Easter Sunday, so joyous that my grandparents were visiting, and so hyped up on Peeps that I couldn't help myself. *I had to twirl.* There is nothing but unrestrained freedom and joy in that picture.

As an adult, I've experienced many moments over the years when I looked at the photo of myself and wondered, when did I stop twirling? Maybe you can relate to the sadness that washed over me when I realized I'd allowed life events to steal my joy. Has something stolen yours?

I believe we were all born to be twirling girls—to live uninhibited and free in this one short life God has given us. Breaking free from debilitating strongholds and false beliefs about our bodies and how we nourish them is how we reclaim the twirling girl that still lives inside each of us. She is inside you, simply waiting for the grown-up you to become aware and set her free.

Once our eyes are opened to how we've been fooled by our culture, the media, a billion-dollar weight loss industry, snake oil salespeople, and the enemy himself, we can't unsee what we've seen. We can't unknow what we now know. Awareness is 99 percent of the battle.

As we heal and reclaim our true selves, we will twirl again, and this freedom has nothing to do with what we weigh. Twirling women come in all shapes and sizes.

We will appear with our arms open, running out into our spacious place of peace. Our singing and twirling will be as worship to the One who brought us there. Our uninhibited joy will become contagious, and others will awaken to what they, too, have kept hidden away. Like the little girls who wished they could twirl with Julie Andrews, they will want to twirl with you, as well.

Imagine a world full of joyful, unencumbered, twirling women proclaiming their healing. Try to picture an army of sisters who do not worry about what they weigh, because they know their God delights in them as they are. The impact to our family, friends, and communities would prove immeasurable. What a beautiful world it would be if we dared to become twirling girls again.

SOUL FITNESS: Strengthening Your Core

When you imagine yourself free, what image comes to mind? Is it a twirling girl or does another picture pop up? Where does this thought come from? A childhood memory? A movie? A painting? A song? Journal why this image is meaningful to you. Go into as much detail as possible. Sit with the image for a while and record your thoughts and feelings.

PRAYER

Heavenly Father, it's hard to picture myself free when I've been tied up for years. Please bring an image to my mind of what freedom could look like for me. Please keep it in front of me when I am discouraged or feel stuck. I choose to accept in faith you are bringing me out into a spacious place and helping me become, because you are delighted in me. Amen.

DAY 26

The LORD is close to the brokenhearted;
he rescues those whose spirits are crushed.

Psalm 34:18 NLT

It's funny how the Lord brings long-forgotten memories to the surface just when you need them. I recently remembered something that happened over fifty years ago.

When I was in late elementary school, my younger brother had a little friend come by to play each day after school. I'll call her Polly. Polly was in the third grade and absolutely adorable. She also had a full head of thick, long hair that often tangled and matted into a large "nest" on the back of her head. It was clean, but it was a mess.

As Polly was the youngest member of a large, chaotic family, her mom probably had no time to brush her daughter's hair. In retrospect, Polly likely loved coming to our house because it was quiet, and my mom always made a snack.

She sat in our family room, cross-legged on the floor, eating cookies with my brother on most days. They'd watch cartoons and nibble before they went outside to play. Even at ten years old, my heart broke at the sight of Polly with all that matted hair. So, I decided to do something about it.

Every day, I would sit behind her on the floor as she munched her cookies while I did my best to untangle the nest.

But my decision didn't immediately translate into implementation. Moving from plan to action took a little convincing for my brother's little friend.

Polly feared I would hurt her and felt a little embarrassed by her hair's condition. But day by day, little by little, I eased her emotions while I used my comb and a soft brush to soothe her strands. When I was done, the tangles were gone, and her hair looked smooth, shiny, and beautiful again. But here's the thing about Polly's situation. She didn't know how to untangle those strands of hair herself—she needed someone to help her. We can identify, because we need assistance too.

Years of neglecting our bodies, of not caring for them properly and ignoring what they truly need, can leave us in a tangle. The problem sometimes becomes too big for us to sort out ourselves. When it does, we need someone to sit with us and help unravel the mess.

We need to understand that it's okay to seek professional help. Yes, God is with you every step of the way. He is truly close to your broken heart, but many times, He sends competent, caring therapists to guide the way when we feel lost.

Seeking help for mental and emotional health does not mean you do not have enough faith or that you are a bad Christian. It doesn't mean you doubt that God can heal you. When Christians are physically sick, they visit their doctor. The same wisdom is needed to care for your mental health and emotional well-being.

A standing appointment each week with an excellent therapist who specializes in women like us will help you move forward. A professional can keep your feet to the fire by holding you accountable. And most of all, they can provide a listening ear and teach you coping skills that provide a safe place to land when emotions hit hard.

As you uncover truth, it will be painful, but with expert support, you will untangle the lies and false beliefs that have kept you stuck. Eventually, the tangles will be eliminated.

I love this saying: *Psychology reveals, but Jesus heals.*

I have experienced the truth of this statement firsthand and believe it with my whole heart. While psychology plays an important role in bringing truth to light and reframes our thinking, Jesus alone brings the healing. Make no mistake—although professional counseling is a beneficial resource, all glory goes to Christ for our recovery from food and body image issues.

Are you at a place where professional assistance may prove your next right step? If so, go to page 132 for some helpful tips on choosing a therapist who is right for you. But do not let pride or fear keep you from seeking support when God may be sending a mental health expert to guide you toward becoming healed.

SOUL FITNESS: Strengthening Your Core

Looking over your past twenty-five days of journaling, what have you discovered so far? What has God revealed to you that you hadn't seen or understood previously? Does seeking professional help from a therapist who specializes in women with body image and food issues seem like the next right step? Why or why not?

PRAYER

Dear Lord, thank you that I live in a time when mental health care no longer carries the stigma it did in times past. I am thankful for the helpers you send to assist us. Please guide me in all decisions I make regarding my mental and emotional health. Thank you for all you have revealed to me, and for helping me become all you want me to be. All glory goes to you. Amen.

DAY 27

*We also have joy with our troubles, because we know
that these troubles produce patience. And patience produces
character, and character produces hope. And this hope will
never disappoint us, because God has poured out his love to fill
our hearts. He gave us his love through the Holy Spirit,
whom God has given to us.*

Romans 5:3–5 NCV

As believers, we know sanctification means inner work will continue until the day we die. We will never attain perfection while on earth, but by applying the Word of God to our lives for growth and maturity, we are *perfected* day by day.

In the past, false promises of dieting success assured us of quick fixes and instant gratification. Fast and immediate are certainly possible with God but are not usually His way.

Lasting change takes time. Especially when it comes to our health, it's important to take the long view and prepare for the long haul. This doesn't mean we won't experience progress early on. God doesn't make us wait— He encourages and cheers us on from the very beginning. From the start, if you look for His handiwork, you will be amazed at what He will do on the inside of you. He is a good and kind Father.

Very early in my healing journey, Pat and I took a long weekend trip to our favorite beach. My grandparents started vacationing there in the 1920s, and we've continued the tradition ever since. This little seaside town is full of boardwalk eateries offering treats I'd enjoyed all my life.

Normally, we did our best to eat all our favorite foods while we were there. The scarcity mindset of a dieter tells you that you'd better have it now, while you can. With so many childhood memories attached, there was a powerful emotional component to having those treats.

This trip was different, though. On the final day of our getaway, I realized I hadn't felt compelled to eat all the treats as I had previously. I enjoyed an ice cream cone at one of our favorite places, and that was that. I realized my scarcity mindset was gone. The emotional charge had disappeared. I didn't have to restrain myself. There was no anxiety or urgency. I knew I could have the caramel popcorn and boardwalk fries the next time we came—if I wanted to.

As for emotional memories of my loved ones, that ice cream cone was my mom's favorite. I realized it had proven enough to satisfy my soul. I didn't need anything else.

My reframed thinking told me there was nothing wrong with emotionally eating from time to time, but on this trip, I didn't need to use food. I reminisced in ways that had nothing to do with familiar flavors. I had other tools in my toolbox now.

When you live in a certain mindset for most of your life, it feels miraculous when you discover God has completely changed how you think. Since our healing begins with our thoughts, these incremental changes helped me appreciate and embrace the long view.

When you've traveled far enough, you realize the road to freedom is not linear. The journey to recovery does not follow a straight path. Expect difficulties. There will be times when other things in your life consume you and demand your focus. All of this is normal. These are the moments when you must remind yourself of the new path you have chosen. Then you can recommit to becoming.

We humans are an impatient lot. Patient waiting seems passive and impossible, but Scripture says the practice is active and produces character (Romans 5:4).

Whether you are walking at an exhilarating pace while God breaks through strongholds one after the other, or on the sluggish stride of taking three steps forward and two backwards, or at a standstill, God is still moving forward with your healing. He is more committed to your wholeness than you are. Transformation can't be rushed.

As you become the woman God desires, let patience do its part. You will learn important truths so vital for your healing. Commit to the long view as He perfects you day by day. In the end, you will experience gratitude for God's teaching as you see the results of His sanctifying inner work.

SOUL FITNESS: Strengthening Your Core

Do you feel like you are on a straight path, or does your progress feel more like hopscotch? If you said the latter, hang on to hope. Christ is developing your character. Describe the pace you are experiencing today. Is God asking you to be patient right now? If so, describe what active patience looks like for you. Give yourself plenty of grace if you need to recommit to the journey. Look for incremental changes you have experienced but may have overlooked. This is a marathon, not a sprint.

PRAYER

Father, it's hard to wait for something I desire so badly. I want to take the shortcut and reach my destination now. Give me the patience I need to take the long view. Please allow me to see the ways I am making progress and becoming who you created me to be. This will give me hope and endurance. Amen.

DAY 28

*And I sent messengers to them, saying, "I am doing a great work
and I cannot come down."*

Nehemiah 6:3 ESV

As you work with the Lord to rebuild and reframe your thinking,
expect naysayers who will try to discourage you from moving forward on the healing path. You should anticipate negativity and prepare to
remain committed.

Our verse today focuses on Nehemiah, a man sent by God to rebuild
the wall of Jerusalem. Once the restoration began, it didn't take long for
naysayers to come out in force, attempting to draw him away from the
mission. They figured if they could lure Nehemiah down from the wall
where he was working, the rebuild would stop in its tracks. Too bad they
didn't figure on Nehemiah's commitment to see the project all the way
through.

With God on his side, Nehemiah refused to come down. He was so
focused on obedience, that he was not deterred by those who bore jeal-
ousy in their hearts. He barely gave the naysayers any of his attention. Due
to Nehemiah's laser-sharp attention to doing what God called him to and
made him for, the restoration was completed.

My dear sister, as you go against the grain of the dieting culture, you will run across friends and family who don't understand. They will evaluate you on how you look and how much weight you've lost instead of how free you are becoming. Some well-meaning people will try to pull you away from where God has led, attempting to convince you to join them on the latest fad diet.

Countless posts and ads on social media will tempt you to doubt the mission. And, sadly, there might be not-so-nice naysayers who will actively work to bring you down. Nehemiah could relate.

When he arrived at Jerusalem to rebuild the wall, Nehemiah knew he was in the center of God's will. This made all the difference for him, and it will for you too. If God has led you to this book and a conviction to move away from the dieting culture, He will give you the focus, strength, and ability to see it through.

When God has taken us to a new place of His choosing, and we are in the center of His will, He doesn't say "good luck" and leave us there. He gives us the power to do what He has asked us to do.

But you can bet that whenever freedom is in the air, the enemy gets nervous. His favorite game is to keep us distracted from God's plans. He does this by selling lies and peddling shame. If he believes you will actually become free, the opposition becomes more intense. You can expect naysayers to come as people and through fiery darts thrown by Satan, God's enemy and ours. Expect it. Plan for it. And stand ready to resist.

You do not owe the opposition any of your time or energy. You don't have to stop and explain yourself to naysayers. You are not obligated to convince anyone of anything. Keep praying. Keep immersing yourself in Scripture. And keep rebuilding your life like Nehemiah rebuilt that wall—one brick at a time.

1. Have confidence in your God.
2. Have confidence in yourself.
3. Have confidence in your calling.

And remember—you are doing a great work. You cannot come down!

SOUL FITNESS: Strengthening Your Core

Make a list of your current naysayers. Next to each one, write an encouraging Scripture that addresses their concerns or criticisms.

For example, my mom thinks I am crazy to stop dieting—"It is dangerous to be concerned with what others think of you, but if you trust the LORD, you are safe" (Proverbs 29:25 GNT).

PRAYER

God, your word encourages me to keep my eyes on you as I become what you desire. You alone are the One who charts my path and reveals your will for my life. Help me to remain patient with loved ones who do not understand what you have called me to do. Help me refuse any negativity that comes my way. Protect me from anything that seeks to pull me off the healing path you've placed me on. Amen.

DAY 29

But You, Lord, are a shield around me,
my glory, and the One who lifts up my head.

Psalm 3:3 HCSB

We're going to spend one more day on shame. It is one of the most debilitating emotions a Christian woman can experience and needs extra attention. As I mentioned before, shame is not from God; however, *holy conviction* is His knock on our heart. They serve very different functions.

Shame is created by Satan to cause maximum damage. Your loving Father convicts to protect you from pain and give you a new life. Shame sends us crawling back into the shadows with our heads bowed low and eyes to the ground. Holy Spirit conviction seeks to draw issues out into the light where they can be dealt with and resolved.

Shame brings dread and hopelessness. God's conviction brings anticipation and hope. Shame brings devastation and isolation. Conviction brings Spirit-filled sorrow that leads to repentance and release. Repentance leads to a new life of deliverance. Just imagine feeling completely free of chronic guilt, anxiety, fear, and shame.

When we sin, our first instinct is usually to go everywhere and to everyone for a rescue before taking it to the Lord. In our search for allies and affirmation, we can sit in sin for a long time without realizing we are out of line. Since we haven't included God, the enemy slinks in to fill the void.

Expect The Shamer to rear his ugly head often while you walk along the healing path. He is dead set against your freedom. He does not want to see you released from the insidious stronghold of unhealthy food and body image behaviors. His goal is to keep you in captivity. He wants you to live a small, isolated, and painful life.

When the Holy Spirit led Jesus into the desert alone (Matthew 4:1–11), God allowed Satan to tempt Him. With each attempted manipulation, Jesus answers the accuser with three simple yet powerful words—"It is written"—and combats Satan's lies by reciting a quote from the living Word of God.

Jesus wielded the sword of the Spirit (Ephesians 6:17). And what was Satan's response? He left. He slunk away as quickly as he slithered in. The enemy's immediate exit proves he's all bluster and no blow. His lies are no match against the spoken Word of God. And Jesus's example, placed in the pages of Scripture for us to model, shows us how to deal with the Prince of Darkness.

But here are some important points you need to keep in mind:

1. You can't quote from a book you haven't read.

2. You can't speak truth you don't believe.

3. And you can't wield a weapon you are not trained to use.

The importance of *knowing* the Word of God and *applying* it to our lives cannot be overstated. If you want to become free, if you want to become the woman you are meant to be, you must read your Bible. By doing so regularly, you will hear directly from your heavenly Father who will speak personally and powerfully to you about your life. The Bible gives us supernatural weapons that repel Satan's emotional lies.

Through the Bible, the Lord shields our way as we walk along the healing path. He places His hand under our chin and lifts our gaze to meet His—and when our eyes lock, we will not see shame mirrored there. Yes, He convicts, but even through that beautiful discipline, you will experience only God's compassion, unconditional love, and grace.

Shame has no place in your heart and soul. Conviction and repentance, however, can heal the wounds carried in your mind, body, and spirit. Today, let's answer the enemy's lies with the Word of God. It is time to declare enough is enough.

SOUL FITNESS: Strengthening Your Core

Make a list of the areas in your life where you feel shame. Next to each, write "It is written" followed by a Scripture that answers the specific shame noted. You can use the search tool at www.biblegateway.com or another biblical resource to help you find appropriate passages related to each specific shame issue. Or simply search for terms like: Scriptures on body image shame, Bible verses about shame, biblical passages on a woman's shame, and so on. Return to these Scriptures often—they will become your lifeline.

PRAYER

Heavenly Father, I am tired from the burden of shame. I believe you do not want me to carry this heaviness any longer. Help me hear your conviction and hide your Word in my heart so I can respond to the enemy and send him packing. Today, I am declaring enough is enough. Thank you, Jesus. Amen.

DAY 30

You say, "I am allowed to do anything"—but not everything is good for you.

1 Corinthians 10:23 NLT

If you've placed dieting on the back burner for a few weeks, you may have noticed there is no cheating, and on-or-off thinking is no longer at play. Ideally, you are nourishing your body with good food three times a day, and if needed, snacks in between. Don't be alarmed if you eat more than you think you should. Give yourself grace. It's perfectly natural to:

- eat more if you've been restricting yourself for a long time.
- allow your body and mind time to adjust.
- want to eat formerly "forbidden foods" since you haven't had them freely for a while. (They aren't forbidden anymore.)
- need time to recover the ability to identify your hunger cues.
- practice processing your emotions instead of running to the fridge.

Don't beat yourself up—these adaptations won't last forever. Everything will eventually settle down if you commit to doing your best at listening and connecting to your body. And if you overdo, it's okay. As you reset, you will not starve yourself. You will not beat yourself up. You will not do anything other than move forward.

Remember, God designed your body to communicate with you. Its voice is still there. Give yourself time to hear it clearly again. You are becoming connected with the pure process God planned.

I've given you many things to think about over the past few weeks. All of them run counter to both the subliminal and overt messages we receive day in and day out, telling us our worth is tied to our outward appearance.

When diet after diet failed me, I cried out to God, "Why can't I eat normally like everyone else?"

Have you asked the same question? Well, here is the answer you've been looking for: *you can eat normally like others.* And do you know what is even better? You will learn to eat in a balanced, natural way that is *normal for you.* You can eat when you're hungry, have ice cream and cake on your birthday, enjoy an appetizer at a party and more—all without rationalizing or explaining. You do not need to make up for special treats. You have perfect autonomy to choose foods you enjoy and in the amount you need.

If you stick with nourishing your body and listening to what it tells you, you will eat purely like many healthy people around the world. I am not saying you should always *eat exactly what others around you are eating*, but you will learn to eat in a way that is best for your unique body.

The days of relapsing, cheating, categorizing food as good or bad, feeling less than, and shaming yourself are over. You are becoming free.

Initially, freedom will feel scary. But decide to live fearlessly. A free woman who's in tune with what foods give her energy and make her feel good will ultimately decide not to eat two buckets of french fries at the carnival. While all foods are on the table and available to her without judgment, she will choose what her wise body guides her to eat. Not all food is beneficial to her well-being. So, she will have a few fries if she wants them, or she will pass. She's not looking for a stomachache. She's looking for peace with food, peace with her body, and peace within herself.

The thread that runs through our broken stories with food and body image is *shame.* The thread that runs through our new story of healing is *grace.* The thread that runs through the story of our ongoing healthy decisions is doing what is *good for you.*

SOUL FITNESS: Strengthening Your Core

Imagine this happening tonight. While you sleep, a miracle occurs. When you awake tomorrow, the shame surrounding your body image and food for so long is gone. It vanished in the darkness. What do you notice that tells you this miracle occurred? What would your life look like from that moment on? How do you feel? List as many changes as you can envision.

PRAYER

Jesus, it feels scary to let go of dieting and trust myself to eat without rules or regulations. Honestly, bondage feels safe to me, even though it's an illusion. I want to replace the thread of shame with the thread of grace and beneficial choices. Help me practice self-compassion as I learn how to live in freedom. Amen.

DAY 31

Jesus turned, and seeing her he said, "Take heart, daughter;
your faith has made you well."

Matthew 9:22 ESV

We are never told her name, but her story is so powerful, it is woven through three of the New Testament Gospels.

This woman had suffered from constant bleeding for twelve long years. In her time, Mosaic Law determined that women who were bleeding, whether it was because of her normal cycle or a more serious medical issue, were ceremonially unclean. There were all kinds of rules and regulations surrounding what that meant and how it was to be handled. But the bottom line was this—she could not live in any way that resembled a normal life.

This woman wasn't allowed to walk freely in the wide-open spaces where everyone else strolled. She existed in a restricted and lonely world. Everywhere she turned, legalism lurked, waiting to judge her. And of course, where there is legalism, there is shame.

She must have felt utterly powerless. On her own, this woman could not find the path to healing, even though she tried. "A woman who had suffered a condition of hemorrhaging for twelve years—a long succession of physicians had treated her, and treated her badly, taking all her money and leaving her worse off than before—had heard about Jesus" (Mark 5:25–26 MSG).

How heartbreaking it must have been to seek a cure repeatedly, only to end up worse off than before she tried the remedy. She must have believed her story would end miserably, with her legacy one of powerlessness and hopelessness.

Does her situation sound familiar to you? It does to me. I, too, have spent much time and money on so-called cures that left me worse than when I started. I got so tired of losing the weight only to cope with heartbreak, disappointment, and shame when I gained the pounds back. I reached a point where I just couldn't go through the disillusionment again. I had tried everything possible—on my own.

In the dark moment of our despair, when we truly come to the end of ourselves, Jesus meets us there. And for our sister in Scripture, the woman with the blood issue, her meeting with Jesus brought the healing she had sought for so long.

She'd heard stories of the rabbi who healed the sick. Maybe she felt she had nothing to lose, so she took an enormous risk. She snuck into a large group of people who had come out to see Jesus.

Remember, this woman was considered unclean, so she was not allowed in public, let alone in a sizable crowd. And in that era, attempting to get near a rabbi was unthinkable for any woman, and even more so for one who had been bleeding for twelve years.

But, even in her weakened state, this woman stepped out in faith. And this time, the outcome was supernaturally different. Her powerlessness instantly disappeared.

> Just then a woman who had been subject to bleeding for twelve years came up behind him and touched the edge of his cloak. She said to herself, "If I only touch his cloak, I will be healed." Jesus turned and saw her. "Take heart, daughter," he said, "your faith has healed you." And the woman was healed at that moment. (Matthew 9:20–22)

What a miracle! The woman who was thought to be incurable, found her cure—not with professionals and experts, but with her Savior. And she received more than one antidote.

In addition to His healing of this woman's physical ailment, Jesus restored her soul. By speaking to an unclean female in public, He demolished the shroud of legalism and shame cast upon her.

As we complete our initial thirty-one days of becoming, I want to encourage you to move forward and reach for Jesus Christ as the perfecter of your healing, just as this dear soul courageously did. Stop trying to resolve your food and body image issues on your own. Quit cowering in fear and shame. It is not too late, and you are not too far gone. Christ *is* your healing and hope.

Take heart, your Savior sees you as you are meant to become, even while He loves you as you are. You may need to read through this book many times over for fresh encouragement and instruction—but Jesus will be behind every word every time. He is patient. He is wise. He is grace. He is freedom. It is He who *will* heal you.

You are still becoming, but you are much closer now than you were a month ago. And a month from now, you will be further on your path to freedom than you are today. Every moment of your transformation is critical to your ultimate outcome, where you finally see yourself as you are intended. A stunning, gorgeous, and absolutely beautiful woman of God.

SOUL FITNESS: Strengthening Your Core

Open your Bible and read the different accounts of the bleeding woman's story in Matthew 9:20–22, Mark 5:25–34, and Luke 8:43–48. If you have time, read them in different translations. Journal about how this woman's story relates to your own.

PRAYER

Dear God, Scripture says: "Jesus did many other things as well. If every one of them were written down, I suppose that even the whole world would not have room for the books that would be written" (John 21:25). Of all the miracles you could have included in the Bible, you chose this woman's story to be one of them. It encourages me as I am still becoming who you want me to be. Thank you and I love you. Amen.

IT'S NOT THE END . . .

If you told me a few years ago that one day I'd be speaking and writing about disordered eating and negative body image, I wouldn't have believed you. Why would I want to voluntarily share the details of such a painful part of my life? And even if I did, who'd want to hear it?

In recent years, I've learned to never underestimate what God can do with a broken woman and her fractured story. The very source of my greatest pain has become one of the greatest joys of my life. I have the honor of telling my sisters about the redeeming and restoring grace of God and maybe to even shine a light, guiding them toward the Healer.

It has been my privilege to share these past thirty-one days with you. I'm trusting that through our time together God has given you specific things to ponder about your own unique broken story. I keep picturing you sitting in a quiet place, hands and heart open, ready to listen to the sweet voice of your Savior.

Scripture speaks often of wide-open spaces in relation to freedom. This imagery has proven especially meaningful to me. I've kept the following passage in front of me for a long time and want to share it with you as we part:

> By entering through faith into what God has always wanted to do for us—set us right with him, make us fit for him—we have it all together with God because of our Master Jesus. And that's not all: We throw open our doors to God and discover at the same moment that he has already thrown open his door to us. We find ourselves standing where we always hoped we might stand—out in the wide open spaces of God's grace and glory, standing tall and shouting our praise. (Romans 5:1–2 MSG)

Friend, be kind to yourself. Give yourself grace. Practice self-compassion. Strengthen your core. Trust your body. And above all else, trust your God. He created you and only He can fix what He has created.

We are in this healing together, and I am cheering you on from the sidelines. We are *still becoming*, and this is only the beginning. What a beautiful, grace-filled place to live in.

With so much love,

Laura

Hunger-Fullness Scale

This is a helpful tool that can be useful as you work on tuning your body's hunger and fullness cues.

1 **Painfully hungry**
Dizzy, stomachache, panicky, urgent – will eat anything.

2 **Extremely hungry**
Hangry. Preoccupied and anxious. All food looks good.

3 **Hungry**
Stomach is empty and growling. Hunger pangs. Time to eat.

4 **Beginning to feel hunger**
Your body is telling you to get ready to eat.

5 **Neutral** Not hungry and not full

6 **Beginning to feel full**
Your body is communicating it's almost time to stop.

7 **Comfortably full**
You have eaten enough to be satiated. Your body feels calm.

8 **Very full**
Beginning to feel uncomfortable. Your body is telling you to stop.

9 **Stuffed**
Clothes feel tight, slightly sick, preoccupied with how full you feel.

10 **Painfully full**
Sick, stomachache, headache, miserable.

Sweet Spot (bracketing items 3–7)

When you start to think about eating or having a meal, check in and ask yourself, where am I on the hunger/fullness scale? What is my body telling me?

When you are finished eating, ask yourself again.

Remember, the goal is not perfection but progress. This takes practice! There will be times when you eat too little or too much. This is normal and will help you understand your hunger cues by trial and error. The goal is to eventually get to a place where you are more consistently staying within the "sweet spot" in the 3 to 7 range.

STEPS TO FIND A MENTAL HEALTH PROVIDER

Personal Preferences: age, gender, cultural background, education, therapeutic focus, faith based.

Questions to Ponder

Do they understand my ethnic and cultural background?

Do they offer a free phone consultation?

Can they assist me in my faith?

Do they specialize in my issue?

Do they take my insurance? If so, do they submit or do I?

Do they offer a sliding scale for payments?

Do they offer telehealth appointments?

Additional Help

National Eating Disorder Association (NEDA) Hotline: (800) 931-2237

If you're depressed, tell someone. Please do not suffer alone, especially if you are suicidal.

If you need immediate emergency services, dial 911.

NOTES

My Story

Geneen Roth, *Women, Food, and God: An Unexpected Path to Almost Everything* (London: Simon & Schuster, 2011), 176–77.

Day 3

Anita A. Johnston, *Eating in the Light of the Moon: How Women Can Transform Their Relationships with Food through Myths, Metaphors & Storytelling* (Carlsbad, CA: Gürze Books, 2000), 17–18.

Strong's Hebrew Lexicon, s.v. "selê," Blue Letter Bible, accessed May 1, 2022, www.blueletterbible.org/lexicon/h5542/kjv/wlc/0-1/.

Day 6

Cristin D. Runfola, Ann Von Holle, Sara E. Trace, Kimberly A. Brownley, Sara M. Hofmeier, Danielle A. Gagne, and Cynthia M. Bulik, "Body Dissatisfaction in Women Across the Lifespan: Results of the UNC-*SELF* and Gender and Body Image (GABI) Studies," *European Eating Disorders Review: The Journal of the Eating Disorders Association*. U.S. National Library of Medicine, January 2013. Last modified January 2013, accessed May 1, 2022, www.ncbi.nlm.nih.gov/pmc/articles/PMC3745223/.

Day 8

"Romans 12:2 Commentary," Precept Austin, July 29, 2017, www.precept austin.org/romans_122#transformed.

Day 9

Oswald Chambers, *My Utmost for His Highest*, ed. James Reimann (1935; Grand Rapids: Discovery House, 1992), March 23.

Day 11

Jan Silvious, *Big Girls Don't Whine: Getting on with the Great Life God Intends* (Nashville: Thomas Nelson, 2003).

Peter Scazzero, *Emotionally Healthy Spirituality: Unleash a Revolution in Your Life in Christ* (Nashville: Thomas Nelson, 2014).

Day 15

Strong's Greek Lexicon, s.v. "ontōs," Blue Letter Bible, accessed May 1, 2022, www.blueletterbible.org/lexicon/g3689/kjv/tr/0-1/.

Day 17

John D. Barry, Douglas Mangum, Derek R. Brown, Michael S. Heiser, Miles Custis, Elliot Ritzema, Matthew M. Whitehead, Michael R. Grigoni, and David Bomar, *Faithlife Study Bible* (Bellingham, WA: Lexham Press, 2012, 2016), Ps 46:10.

Day 19

"Step Four," Big Book Recovery, www.bigbookrecovery.com, accessed May 4, 2022, www.bigbookrecovery.com/index.php/step-four.

Day 20

Carolyn Custis James, "A Forgotten Legacy—Eve," in *Lost Women of the Bible: The Women We Thought We Knew* (Grand Rapids: Zondervan, 2008), 35–36.

Day 25

Pat Bauer, "The Sound of Music," Britannica, www.britannica.com/topic /The-Sound-of-Music-film-by-Wise.

Laurence Maslon, "The Charts Are Alive with *The Sound of Music*," Rodgers & Hammerstein, August 20, 2020, https://rodgersand hammerstein.com/the-sound-of-music-the-charts-are-alive-with-the-sound-of-music/.

ABOUT THE AUTHOR

Laura Acuña is a speaker, author, life coach, and podcast host. She exudes warmth, fun, and authenticity, passionately sharing truths gleaned through God's Word and lessons learned along the way. Her passion is to help women move from where they are now to where they want to be—healed, whole, and in a deeper walk with Jesus. Married to Pat, they are the parents of three sons and one daughter-in-love. Their first grandchild (finally a girl!) arrived in 2021.

Laura is a graduate of Liberty University where she earned a degree in Christian counseling and a minor in biblical studies, summa cum laude. She's the cofounder of Sisters in Faith Ministries, a non-profit ministry to women in her area. Laura has served as a women's ministry leader in various capacities for over twenty-three years. She lives in Damascus, Maryland, and serves at Damascus Road Community Church.

You can find Laura at www.Laura-Acuna.com, on the *Still Becoming* podcast, and most social media platforms.

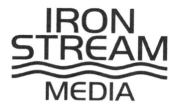

If you enjoyed this book, will you consider sharing the message with others?

Let us know your thoughts. You can let the author know by visiting or sharing a photo of the cover on our social media pages or leaving a review at a retailer's site. All of it helps us get the message out!

Email: info@ironstreammedia.com

  @ironstreammedia

Iron Stream, Iron Stream Fiction, Iron Stream Kids, Brookstone Publishing Group, and Life Bible Study are imprints of Iron Stream Media, which derives its name from Proverbs 27:17, "As iron sharpens iron, so one person sharpens another." This sharpening describes the process of discipleship, one to another. With this in mind, Iron Stream Media provides a variety of solutions for churches, ministry leaders, and nonprofits ranging from in-depth Bible study curriculum and Christian book publishing to custom publishing and consultative services.

For more information on ISM and its imprints, please visit
IronStreamMedia.com

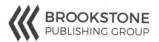